BOOK ENDOMORPH

TABLE OF CONTENTS

Introduction	**7**
Understanding the Endomorph Body Type	7
The Importance of Customized Strategies for Health and Fitness	8
Chapter 1: Foundations of Endomorph Wellness	**9**
Endomorph Body Type	9
Advantages of Being an Endomorph	10
Chapter 2: Goal Setting for Endomorphs	**11**
Defining Your Wellness Objectives	11
S.M.A.R.T. Goals for Endomorphs	11
Tracking Progress and Sustaining Motivation	12
Chapter 3: Nutritional Strategies for Endomorphs	**14**
Essential Nutrients for Endomorphs	14
3 Myths Blocking Your Endomorph Fat Loss	19
5 Food Types You Need to Say Goodbye To	20
Effective Calorie Tracking Techniques	23
Chapter 4: Meal Planning and Culinary Inspiration	**25**
Organizing Weekly Meals for Endomorphs	25
Guidelines Meal Plan	26
Breakfast Recipes	27
Spinach and Feta Omelet	27
Almond Butter Berry Smoothie	28
Greek Yogurt Parfait	29
Scrambled Tofu	29
Cottage Cheese Bowl	30
Protein Pancakes	31
Egg Muffins	31
Chia Seed Pudding	32
Avocado Toast	33
Turkey Sausage and Veggie Skillet	33
Mixed Berry Oatmeal	34
Avocado and Salmon Bagel	35
Peanut Butter Banana Smoothie	35
Veggie Breakfast Hash	36
Egg and Spinach Breakfast Wrap	36
Alternatives for Busy People	38
Avocado Egg Toast	38
Nutty Greek Yogurt Delight	38
Spinach Banana Protein Shake	38
Lunch Recipes	38
Chicken Quinoa Salad	39
Turkey Avocado Wrap	39

Beef and Broccoli Stir-Fry	40
Lentil Soup	41
Tuna Salad Stuffed Bell Peppers	41
Shrimp Avocado Salad	42
Grilled Salmon and Asparagus	43
Sweet Potato and Black Bean Bowl	43
Mushroom and Spinach Frittata	44
Quinoa and Vegetable Stuffed Peppers	45
Chickpea Salad Sandwich	45
Asian Chicken Lettuce Wraps	46
Alternatives for Busy People	47
Tuna in Lettuce Cups	47
Chickpea Veggie Toss	47
Cheese and Turkey Pinwheels	47
Dinner Recipes	48
Baked Cod with Roasted Veggies	48
Zucchini Noodles with Turkey Meatballs	49
Stuffed Acorn Squash	49
Grilled Chicken and Vegetable Kebabs	50
Beef Stew	51
Cauliflower Crust Pizza	51
Spaghetti Squash Bolognese	52
Pork Tenderloin with Green Beans	53
Chicken Fajita Bowl	53
Salmon Patty Burgers	54
Garlic Herb Roasted Chicken and Root Vegetables	54
Baked Lemon Pepper Fish with Green Beans	55
Coconut Curry Vegetable Lentil Stew	55
Spicy Ground Turkey and Quinoa Stuffed Peppers	56
Greek Chickpea and Vegetable Salad	57
Alternatives for Busy People	58
Salmon Quick Fix	58
Beef Spinach Sauté	58
Scrambled Egg & Avocado Plate	58
Healthy Snacks and Sides Recipes	59
Greek Yogurt with Berries	59
Hummus and Veggie Sticks	59
Almond Butter and Apple Slices	59
Quinoa Salad	59
Roasted Chickpeas	60
Dining out and social eating	60
Chapter 5: A 28-Day Nutritional Plan for Endomorphs	**62**
5 Nutritional Notes to Keep in Mind	62
Week 1 Plan	63

Week 2 Plan	66
Week 3 Plan	70
Week 4 Plan	73
Chapter 6: Physical Activity Guidelines for Endomorphs	**77**
The Role of Exercise in Endomorph Weight Management	77
The 4 Main Principles for Endomorph Fitness Routines	78
Exercise Timing for Endomorphs	81
Chapter 7: Comprehensive Workout Programs	**82**
List of Exercises and How to Perform Them	82
• LEGS	82
Squats	82
Glute Bridge	83
Lunges	84
Step-Ups	84
Wall Sit	85
Deadlifts	85
Kettlebell Swing	86
• UPPER BODY	88
Push-Ups	88
Barbell Rows	88
Bench Press	89
Pull-Ups	90
Overhead Press	90
• CORE	91
Plank	91
Side Plank	91
Russian Twist	92
Leg Raises	92
• CARDIO	93
HIIT Sprints	93
Jump Rope	93
Rowing Machine	94
Burpees	94
How to Warm-Up and Cool-Down Effectively	95
A 12-Week Fitness Schedule for Endomorphs	97
Week 1	99
• Session 1 - Strength Training session	99
• Session 2 - HIIT session	99
• Session 3 - Strength Training session	100
• Session 4 - HIIT session	100
• Session 5	101
Week 2	102
• Session 1 - Strength Training session	102
• Session 2 - HIIT session	102

- Session 3 - Strength Training session … 103
- Session 4 - HIIT session … 103
- Session 5 … 104

Week 3 … 105
- Session 1 - Strength Training session … 105
- Session 2 - HIIT session … 105
- Session 3 - Strength Training session … 106
- Session 4 - HIIT session … 106
- Session 5 … 107

Week 4 … 108
- Session 1 - Strength Training session … 108
- Session 2 - HIIT session … 108
- Session 3 - Strength Training session … 109
- Session 4 - HIIT session … 109
- Session 5 … 110

Week 5 … 111
- Session 1 - Strength Training session … 111
- Session 2 - HIIT session … 111
- Session 3 - Strength Training session … 112
- Session 4 - HIIT session … 112
- Session 5 … 113

Week 6 - Deload Week … 114
- Session 1 - Strength Training session … 114
- Session 2 - HIIT session … 114

Between HIIT Sprints and Jumping Rope take 2-3 minutes break.
- Session 3 - Strength Training session (decrease load or reps here no sets) 115
- Session 4 - HIIT session … 115
- Session 5 … 116

Week 7 … 117
- Session 1 - Strength Training session … 117
- Session 2 - HIIT session … 117
- Session 3 - Strength Training session … 118
- Session 4 - HIIT session … 118
- Session 5 … 119

Week 8 … 120
- Session 1 - Strength Training session … 120
- Session 2 - HIIT session … 120
- Session 3 - Strength Training session … 121
- Session 4 - HIIT session … 121
- Session 5 … 122

Week 9 … 123
- Session 1 - Strength Training session … 123
- Session 2 - HIIT session … 123
- Session 3 - Strength Training session … 124

- Session 4 - HIIT session ... 124
- Session 5 ... 125

Week 10 ... 126
- Session 1 - Strength Training session ... 126
- Session 2 - HIIT session ... 126
- Session 3 - Strength Training session ... 127
- Session 4 - HIIT session ... 127
- Session 5 ... 128

Week 11 ... 129
- Session 1 - Strength Training session ... 129
- Session 2 - HIIT session ... 129
- Session 3 - Strength Training session ... 130
- Session 4 - HIIT session ... 130
- Session 5 ... 131

Week 12- Deload Week ... 132
- Session 1 - Strength Training session ... 132
- Session 2 ... 132
- Session 3 - Strength Training session ... 132
- Session 4 -Between Rowing Machine and Burpees take 2-3 minutes break. 133
- Session 5 ... 133

Chapter 8: Rest, Recovery, and Rejuvenation ... **134**
Integrating Rest into Your Wellness Routine ... 134
Enhancing Recovery with Practical Strategies ... 135
Stress Management and Sleep Improvement Techniques ... 136

Chapter 9: Easy-to-Read Guide on Supplemental Support for Endomorphs ... **137**
FAQs ... **140**
Conclusion ... **143**

INTRODUCTION

Understanding the Endomorph Body Type

Understanding your body type, especially if you're an endomorph, is a big step to become healthier and fitter. I'm a health and nutrition coach, and I've helped lots of people who are endomorphs. Endomorphs usually have a solid and round body. They find it easy to gain weight but hard to lose it. While this might sound less than ideal, understanding it can help you turn it to your advantage—yes, there are advantages!

Endomorphs are often very strong and can do well in activities that need a lot of power. However, because their bodies work a bit slower in burning calories, therefore having a smart plan for nutrition and exercise is crucial. In fact, you cannot expect to eat junk food or exercise sporadically like an ectomorph (people that find it difficult to gain weight and have fast metabolism) might do and expect not to gain body fat.

For endomorphs to be in their best shape, you must focus on two things: **what you eat** and **how you exercise**.

For eating, it's all about choosing foods that help your body work better. We won't get into the details here, but we'll dive deep as there are chapters tailored for diet, guidelines, recipes as well as a **28-Day Nutritional Guideline**). The same goes for exercise. There's a mix of workouts that are just right for endomorphs, making sure you get strong and burn calories efficiently with a weekly training plan that works on all areas. We'll cover all the best exercises for you in upcoming chapters, as well as providing you with an **Easy-to-follow 12-Week Plan**.

In short, this book will guide you through everything about eating right and exercising that fits you best. Additionally, I will dispel some myths about endomorphs and offer other hacks you can incorporate into your lifestyle to further enhance your results!

The Importance of Customized Strategies for Health and Fitness

Creating a health and fitness plan that's tailored just for you is crucial because everyone's body and needs are unique. Here are a few reasons why personalized plans work best.

First, **personal plans keep you engaged**. When your exercise and diet feel like they're designed just for you, they tend to be more enjoyable. This means you're more likely to stick with it because it fits into your life perfectly without needing to make extra efforts.

Second, **a plan made for you considers your own health and goals**. If you're dealing with specific health issues or you have certain fitness goals in mind, a generalized approach is unlikely to work. A custom plan for endomorphs will ensure you're doing what's best for your body, helping you get better results effectively. This is the closest you'll get to an individualized plan, with lots of recipes endomorph-friendly and proven workouts that create lasting results for your body type.

Third, **a customized plan can change as you do**, which is key for continuous progress. As you get stronger and more fit, what you need changes. A plan that can change with you helps you keep getting better and stops you from feeling stuck. I made a 12-week plan because it gives you plenty of time to see how much you can improve. I think 28 days is just too short for most people to really see changes.

To recap, having effective nutritional and training plans keeps you motivated, pushes you to reach your goals, and keeps you on track. I am a big believer that fitness goals can be achieved more effectively with this personalized approach.

Chapter 1:
FOUNDATIONS OF ENDOMORPH WELLNESS

Endomorph Body Type

Let's explain in detail what an endomorph body type is. If you find out you're an endomorph, that means you have a body type that's naturally strong and suited for strength-based sports, like lifting weights. People with this body type often stand out in activities such as in weightlifting competitions or CrossFit challenges (not sure it's you, but just letting you know you have a great foundation for these sports!).

Endomorphs have a sturdy, broad build, and even when they're very fit, they tend to have a fuller shape with wider hips and waist. This is regardless of gender.

The main disadvantage is that you might find it harder to keep a low level of body fat (under 13-15% for men and 20% for women) even if you're active or in good shape. This is because your metabolism tends to be slightly slower than average, making you feel less energetic and athletic once your diet is not on point.

The key for endomorphs is about understanding your strengths and how to make them work for you, without focusing too much on specific diets or workouts just yet. This introduction is designed to prepare you for getting clear about the best ways to eat and exercis

WHAT'S MY BODY TYPE?

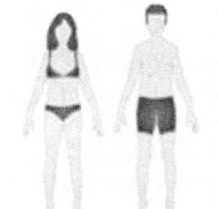

ECTOMORPH
- SMALL "DELICATE" FRAME AND BONE STRUCTURE
- FLAT CHEST
- THIN
- LEAN MUSCLE MASS
- FAST METABOLISM
- FIND IT HARD TO GAIN WEIGHT
- CLASSIC "HARDGAINER"
- SMALL SHOULDERS

MESOMORPH
- ATHLETIC
- WELL DEFINED MUSCLES
- STRONG
- GAIN MUSCLE EASILY
- GAINS FAT MORE EASILY THAN ECTOMORPH
- RECTANGULAR SHAPED BODY
- GENERALLY HARD BODY

ENDOMORPH
- MUSCLES NOT SO DEFINED
- FINDS IT HARD TO LOSE FAT
- "STOCKY" BUILD
- SOFT AND ROUND BODY
- IS GENERALLY SHORT
- ROUND PHYSIQUE
- SLOW METABOLISM
- GAIN MUSCLE AND FAT VERY EASILY

Advantages of Being an Endomorph

Do not get demotivated though! You can get great results fitness wise. Here are the main advantages you have that probably didn't know:

- **Lower Risk of Osteoporosis** Thanks to the body structure, endomorphs tend to need a small amount of consistent exercise to strengthen bones and connective tissue compared to other body types. In fact, endomorphs have less risk of osteoporosis on average.
  (Yes, you need more exercise compared to other body types to keep your weight controlled but less exercise in terms of strength-development)

- **Strength Advantages**: The endomorph's additional mass naturally facilitates muscular development, making them great at strength-required sports, as we previously mentioned.

- **Health Misconceptions**: Being an endomorph doesn't automatically mean poor health like high cholesterol or blood pressure. It's possible to be healthy regardless of body type. It's actually the most advantageous body type if you're serious about your health and nutrition!
  Exercise and diet somewhat consistently and you won't have to worry about being fragile, weak or at risk for osteoporosis (unless it runs in the family).

Chapter 2:
GOAL SETTING FOR ENDOMORPHS

Defining Your Wellness Objectives

Determining your goals clearly is similar to putting points on a map of your journey toward a better you. For endomorphs, **specificity is essential**. A good goal would be, for instance, "*I want to run a 5K in six months to improve my stamina.*" or *"I want to lose 5kg before my friend's wedding in 8 weeks"* These objectives are specific and provide you with a clear goal and direction. However, a goal as vague as "*I want to get fit*" doesn't really provide you with much guidance. It's overly general and leaves out important details like what "fit" actually entails and how to recognize it. As a rule, make your goal as specific as possible.

John is a good example. He is a friend of mine and had a goal to finish a 5K run, not just to "get in shape." His training was directed by this particular goal, which gave his workouts direction and purpose (in his case we thought that an approach of a mix between long runs, interval training and a bit of strength training was best). In three months of consistent hard work he did it. And as a result he got in the best shape of his life.

Recap: Make sure that your goals are specific and should motivate you, fitting into your life in a way that is both gratifying and doable!

S.M.A.R.T. Goals for Endomorphs

Making goals SMART (Specific, Measurable, Achievable, Relevant, Time-bound) turns wishful thinking into achievable objectives. "*To add three strength training sessions per week into my routine for the next 12 weeks*' ' could be a very good goal for an endomorph. It has a deadline, is realistic, quantifiable, and directly linked to enhancing body composition aka being fitter.

On the other hand, *"I want to lose weight fast"* might be a poorly defined goal. Because it doesn't specify how much weight to lose, how you are going to lose it and how long to lose it.

This goal is not only unrealistic but also potentially unhealthy for an endomorph. In fact, aiming for a rapid weight loss can be harmful and unsustainable (you might have tried it already).

A good example is my wife's sister Sarah. Her strategy of progressively adding weights week by week to her exercise routine is an excellent example of a SMART goal. She didn't just jump right into heavy lifting; instead, she started small, making her goal attainable and positioning herself for success. *Note*: Lifting extremely heavy weights right away could cause injuries, joint discomfort or burnout.

Tracking Progress and Sustaining Motivation

Monitoring your development is crucial. When it comes to endomorphs who may want to lose a few pounds, weight alone doesn't always tell the whole story. Merely concentrating on the scale would be a poor example of tracking progress as you would not know if you are losing body fat or muscle mass.

Here are two ways to track your progress effectively:

- **Body Composition**

Do body composition every 4 to 6 weeks. This way you are sure whether you are going in the right direction or there are some adjustments to be made. Also, try to always do it in the same condition. In fact, if you do them one day on an empty stomach and the next check after 4-6 weeks in the evening after dinner, the results would not be accurate.

- **Body Measurement**

If you do not have access to it, you can take measurements of your weight, waist, thighs and arms (make sure to always take the same points, without going an inch higher or lower). Measure them every 4 weeks and see them changing.

Ideally you'd want your waist to slim down a lot while arms and thighs depend on your physique. Some people do not accumulate excessive body fat in those areas, so slimming down these areas would mainly result in muscle mass loss.

Here are two ways you can sustain motivation for long period of time:

- **Rewarding small successes**

I can assure you that rewarding minor successes is essential for maintaining motivation.Just make sure that those rewards do not have a negative impact on your goals. Let's make an example:

If you buy yourself new running shoes as a positive and fitting reward for working out consistently for a month, this is a great reward. On the other hand, rewarding yourself with a big, unhealthy meal after working out can backfire and undermine your efforts.

- **Having an accountability partner**

If you struggle with motivation and staying consistent, getting involved in a community of support can help you stay accountable and offer encouragement. Sharing setbacks and victories reduces the sense of isolation during the journey. On the other hand, trying to do it by yourself can be really tough and might make you want to give up, especially when little problems pop up. Like, if you miss a few workouts because you're sick or too busy, or if you don't stick to your eating plan for a couple of days, some people think they "failed" and definitely give up on their fitness.

Chapter 3
NUTRITIONAL STRATEGIES FOR ENDOMORPHS

Essential Nutrients for Endomorphs

For endomorphs, knowing exactly what to eat is paramount. In order to optimize health, and support the specific needs of their body type, it's important to understand the significance of critical nutrients, where to get them and the potential issues of deficiencies.

Here I am going to explain what are the essential nutrients and some food that you could consume (in the next chapter you will see over 80 recipes and a nutritional plan)

- ***Protein***

In addition to helping endomorphs build lean mass, protein helps them repair and grow muscles, thereby increasing metabolism. A good standard is 1g of protein for each pound of weight. Let's say you weight 180 pounds, you should aim to consume 180g/protein daily

Here are some good plant-based options such:

Food	Protein for 100g
Black Beans	21g
Tempeh	19g
Chickpeas	19g
Lentils	9g
Tofu	8g
Quinoa	4.4g

While good sources of lean protein animal-based are:

Food	Protein for 100g
Chicken Breast	33g
Turkey Breasts	30g
Lean Beef	26-32g
Tuna	25g
Salmon	22g
Cod	17g
Egg White	11g

Why do you have to consume them daily?

The lack of protein in your diet can lead to decreased muscle recovery post-exercise, which can result in a suboptimal body composition overtime (in fact, you won't maximize your muscle mass and burn body fat as you would have if you ate enough protein).

Slowing down your metabolism is the last thing you want as an endomorph as it will become very easy to store far that way.

- ***Fiber***

Fiber plays an integral role in maintaining digestive health and keeping us full. Men should aim for 30-35g daily. Women should aim for 20-25 g daily.There are many foods that naturally contain fiber, here is a list of the main ones.

Food	Fiber for 100g
Chia Seeds and Flaxseeds	34g
Chickpeas	12g
Whole Oats	11g
Beans	10g
Avocado	6-7g
Berries	5-6g
Leafy Greens	3g
Quinoa	3g

Why do you have to consume them daily?

Fiber slows digestion and makes us feel full, so low-fiber diets can make us hungry more frequently. Due to this, we can end up overeating - and those chips and cookies won't be what we crave.

- ***Healthy Fats***

These fats are essential to maintaining hormonal balance and steady energy. You should assume 20 to 35% of total calories from fats (so anywhere between 45 and 75g per day on average).

Prime healthy sources are the following:

Note: *these are considered healthy sources as they are relatively low in saturated fats and high in monounsaturated ones.*

Food	Fats in 100g
Extra virgin olive oil	100g
Macadamia nuts	76g
Walnuts	65g
Dark chocolate	43g
Chia seeds	31g
Egg Yolk	27g
Avocado	15g

Why do you have to consume them daily?

Lacking sufficient healthy fats in your diet could negatively impact your metabolic health and mood stability. Indeed, they are instrumental in preserving hormonal harmony, ensuring the body remains in a balanced state.

- ***Complex Carbohydrates***

Provide a steady energy release without the sugar highs and crashes that simple carbs are known for. Once you eat the daily dose of proteins and fats, the rest of your daily calories should come from carbohydrates.

Good examples are listed below.

Food	Carbohydrates in 100g
Oats	55g
Whole-grain pasta	41g
Barley	28g
Brown rice	26g
Quinoa	21g
Sweet potatoes	20g

Why do you have to consume them daily?

Overly restricting carbs can lead to low energy levels, which could have you cutting your workouts short. A big mistake people make is to avoid carbs. You need them, just eat the right type!

- **Vitamins and Minerals**

A varied diet generally meets these nutritional needs, no matter your body type. However, it's always important to make sure to get the nutrients that help to support your body. Here are the main ones and next to them some foods that can help you meet your nutritional needs

Vitamins and Minerals	Recommended Food	Why are they important?
Iron	Red meat, seafood, beans, lentils	Essential for making hemoglobin, which carries oxygen in the blood, and supports your energy levels.
Calcium	Milk, yogurt, green vegetables, almond milk, soy milk, rice milk	Vital for bone health, muscle function, nerve signaling, and heart health.
Vitamin D	Salmon, mackerel, sardines and sun *(very important)*	crucial for calcium absorption, bone health, immune function, and reducing inflammation.
Potassium	Bananas, spinach and avocados	Regulates fluid balance, muscle contractions, and nerve signals, and reduces blood pressure risk.

Zinc	Oysters, red meat and lentils	Important for immune function and aids wound healing.
Magnesium	Dark chocolate, almonds and quinoa	Contribute to optimal muscle and nerve function, energy production, and vital for heart health and bone strength.

Get those on the regular, as ignoring those micronutrients means less energy, longer illnesses, and a slower metabolism. Without these, your body isn't as capable of that tight-roping act as it wants to be.

Key signs of vitamin and mineral deficiencies are listed here, though they may indicate other issues too:

Vitamins and Minerals	Common Symptoms of Lacking
Iron	Fatigue, weakness, pale skin, cold hands and feet, headaches, brittle nails.
Calcium	Weak bones, numbness, fatigue, nail and skin problems, abnormal heart rhythms.
Vitamin D	Bone pain, muscle weakness, mood changes, increased risk of fractures, impaired wound healing.
Potassium	Muscle cramps, digestive problems, heart palpitations, breathing difficulties, mood changes.
Zinc	Weak immune system, hair loss, diarrhea, eye and skin lesions, loss of appetite, slow growth.
Magnesium	Osteoporosis, high blood pressure, irregular heartbeat, asthma, sleep issues.

In addition, I'd like to mention the importance of Omega-3 fatty acids. They are noteworthy for their anti-inflammatory properties and support for brain health.Good fonts are walnuts, flaxseeds, hemp seeds, salmon and sardines.

3 Myths Blocking Your Endomorph Fat Loss

As an endomorph trying to lose weight, it's easy to get caught up in a lot of advice that makes it feel like you're not going to be able to meet your goals. Let's clear the air about three big myths about the endomorph diet:

1. "You're Stuck With Your Body Forever" - Not True!

You've heard it before — people say if you're an endomorph, then you're stuck with it and can't change how your body looks. But you know what? That's completely and utterly false.

Just follow a tailored endomorph diet, eating the right food and doing the right workouts for a consistent period of time and you'll see how your body will change. Remember that you can do it!

2. "Endomorphs Have to Work Harder Than Others" - That's Not the Whole Story.

When you feel like you have to do 10 times as much as anyone else to lose an ounce, that's so frustrating. But you don't need to work harder, you need to work smarter. We all have our challenges: Maybe as an endomorph, you watch your caloric intake slightly more than another body type. But with some good planning and finding your personal plan, it doesn't have to feel impossible. This is a myth that might make you feel like giving up, especially when life gets a little too real.

3. "You Must Eat Super Low Carbs to Lose Weight" - There's More to It.

There's a lot of talk about whittling carbs way down or going keto-level low. The problem is, with less carbs, some people will lose weight for a little while…but then it stalls, it's not the only way, and you can't maintain it for a long time. Eating a variety of types of foods, as I showed you before (and more detailed in the next chapter with over 80 recipes) is oftentimes the better plan of action. The ideal diet is one that suits you well, encompasses a variety of foods, and is sustainable beyond just a two-week annual attempt before discontinuation.

Make sure you don't fall for these myths! Yes, your habits initiate how much priority your body will give to fat-storing, but you can change, you don't have to work miserably hard to do it and you don't need to go carbless for it.

> If you start the following nutritional and fitness plan, and stick to it, you will reach your goals, no question!

5 Food Types You Need to Say Goodbye To

Listed below are five categories of foods that you should avoid, or at least drastically reduce, for weight loss:

Steer Clear of Highly Processed Foods

Fast food, packaged snacks, and sugary drinks are full of "empty" calories, rich in sugar and unhealthy fats. When you eat these foods, you are slowly destroying your body. Over time, your blood sugar spikes, which causes your body to store fat,.These grab-and-go meals may be easy to find and tasty, but they'll ruin your weight loss efforts.

Healthier Alternatives: Consider opting for homemade meals, such as grilled chicken or fish, fresh vegetables, and whole grains like quinoa or brown rice. Snack on fruits, nuts, or yogurt instead of reaching for packaged snacks, and choose water, herbal teas, or homemade smoothies over sugary beverages.

Why is this important for endomorphs? Endomorphs have a slower metabolism, making it easier for them to store fat, especially when consuming high-calorie, nutrient-poor processed foods. By avoiding these, you can make sure not to slow down your progress.

Limit Foods High in Saturated and Trans Fats

Fried foods, fatty meats, and high-fat dairy products are high in saturated and trans fats, which not only "help" to increase body fat but also increase your risk of heart disease.

Healthier Alternatives: Consider baking, grilling, or steaming your meals instead of frying. Opt for lean protein sources like poultry, fish, and plant-based proteins to replace fatty meats. Swap high-fat dairy products (especially if they cause you digestive problems) for their low-fat or plant-based alternatives, such as almond milk, Greek yogurt or coconut yogurt.

Why is this important for endomorphs? Endomorphs, as mentioned numerous times by now, are predisposed to storing fat more easily, and saturated and trans fats contribute significantly to this issue. They also increase the risk of heart disease.

Cut Down on Added Sugars

It's easy to over consume added sugars found in sweets like candy, cookies, and cakes. These not only contribute to weight gain by providing excessive calories but also by promoting fat storage, as mentioned before.

Imagine working hard in the gym and ruining your training by coming back home and eating cookies? Would that be a smart move? I am sure you know it's not!

Healthier Alternatives: Turn to natural sources of sweetness such as fruits. Berries, apples, and oranges, for example, can provide the sweet taste you like along with beneficial fibers, vitamins, and minerals. Dark chocolate with a high cocoa content is a good food too; make sure to not overeat it and that it is at least 80% dark chocolate (and eat it in moderation, obviously).

Why is this important for endomorphs? By reducing intake of added sugars and opting for natural sweetness sources like fruits, you can avoid counteracting their weight loss efforts and support a healthier metabolic profile. This will not serve you only for losing weight effectively but also to feel more alive, energetic and have less risk of cardiovascular diseases.

Change White Bread and Refined Grains for Whole Grains

White bread and other refined grains might be staple foods, but they're low in nutrients and can lead to blood sugar spikes, which as you probably know by now, facilitate fat storage in your body.

Healthier Alternatives: See what works for you. Incorporating whole grains such as brown rice, quinoa, and whole wheat or rye bread into your diet can be a beneficial switch. These healthier alternatives offer a wealth of fiber, which aids in satiety, helps manage hunger, and supports stable blood sugar levels, contributing to better metabolic health.

Why is this important for endomorphs? Refined grains and white bread lead to blood sugar spikes, which is not great if you aim at losing weight but also can make you feel lethargic and sleepy during the day.

Moderate Your Alcohol Intake

Alcohol contains empty calories (it means it has calories but they do not have any nutritional value) and it also messes with your hormone levels and slows down your metabolism, making weight loss harder. Especially when you start your weight loss journey, cutting down or even eliminating alcohol for a while is a great choice.

Healthier Alternatives: Sparkling water with a splash of lemon (optional), herbal teas, or infused waters can not only help in avoiding the calorie intake from alcohol but also give you a different taste that probably still water does not give you.

Why is this important for endomorphs? Alcohol has also a negative effect on hormone levels and metabolism can make weight loss even more challenging for endomorphs.

Incorporate these tips into your daily routine and watch as your body transforms. You'll feel better, have more energy for workouts and daily tasks, and bid farewell to the old you!

Recap

Foods to Avoid	What to Eat Instead
Packaged Snacks and Sugary Drinks	Grilled Chicken or Fish, Fresh Vegetables, Quinoa, Brown Rice, Homemade Smoothies
Fried foods, fatty meats, and high-fat dairy products	Baking, grilling, or steaming your meals. Poultry, Fish, and plant-based proteins. Almond milk, Soy milk, Rice milk, Greek yogurt or coconut yogurt.
Candy, Cookies and Cakes	Fruits
White Bread and Refined Grains	Brown Rice, Quinoa, and Whole Wheat or Rye Bread
Alcohol	Sparkling Water, Herbal Teas and Infused Water

Effective Calorie Tracking Techniques

These are three effective techniques you can start implementing today (pick the one you like the most):

1. Keeping a Food Journal

A food journal is much more than just another weight loss trick. The simple act of writing down what you eat makes you more aware of what you're eating, and prevents you from mindlessly munching. So, for your breakfast of eggs and toast, you would write down "Large egg fried in 1/2 tsp butter, 1 slice wheat bread".

Ideally you would also write the calories you consume, such as "Large egg fried in 1/2 tsp butter, 74 calories" and "1 slice wheat bread, 70 calories" for a total of 144 calories.

For Beginners:

If starting a food journal just feels like too much, get a little less detailed. Start by writing down just one meal a day, presumably the healthy one. As you get more comfortable with the process, the difficulties of doing it for every meal and snack won't seem so daunting.

2. Using Calorie Counter Apps

Apps like MyFitnessPal make it easy to keep track of your diet. You can search for the foods you eat and quickly add them to your daily log, or scan barcodes for pre-packaged foods. You'll also get a nutritional breakdown, showing you the protein, fat, carbs, and more that you're consuming, which is great for making sure you're getting a well-rounded diet.

For Beginners:

If you are unfamiliar with calorie counter apps, start by logging one meal a day or your snacks. This way, you can get comfortable with the app's features without feeling overwhelmed. Overtime, you can gradually start to add more meals until you are tracking your entire day's intake.

3. Learning About Serving Sizes

Learning on serving sizes naturally helps us know what we eat and counting the calories. A palm-size portion of meat and a fist-sized serving of veggies is a good place to start. However, there are other visual cues to remember, and the key is staying balanced.

Remember, we're trying to <u>eat healthier without counting every single calorie</u>. By visualizing, it does make it easier to manage how much you actually eat and not overeat.

For Beginners:

Lee suggests starting with one type of food if you're new to estimating serving sizes. Let's say you want to know how much protein to eat. Make a mental note of any protein (a few slices of turkey, a hamburger patty, a small chicken breast). Over time you will figure out visually how much carbs, fat and protein you should be consuming.

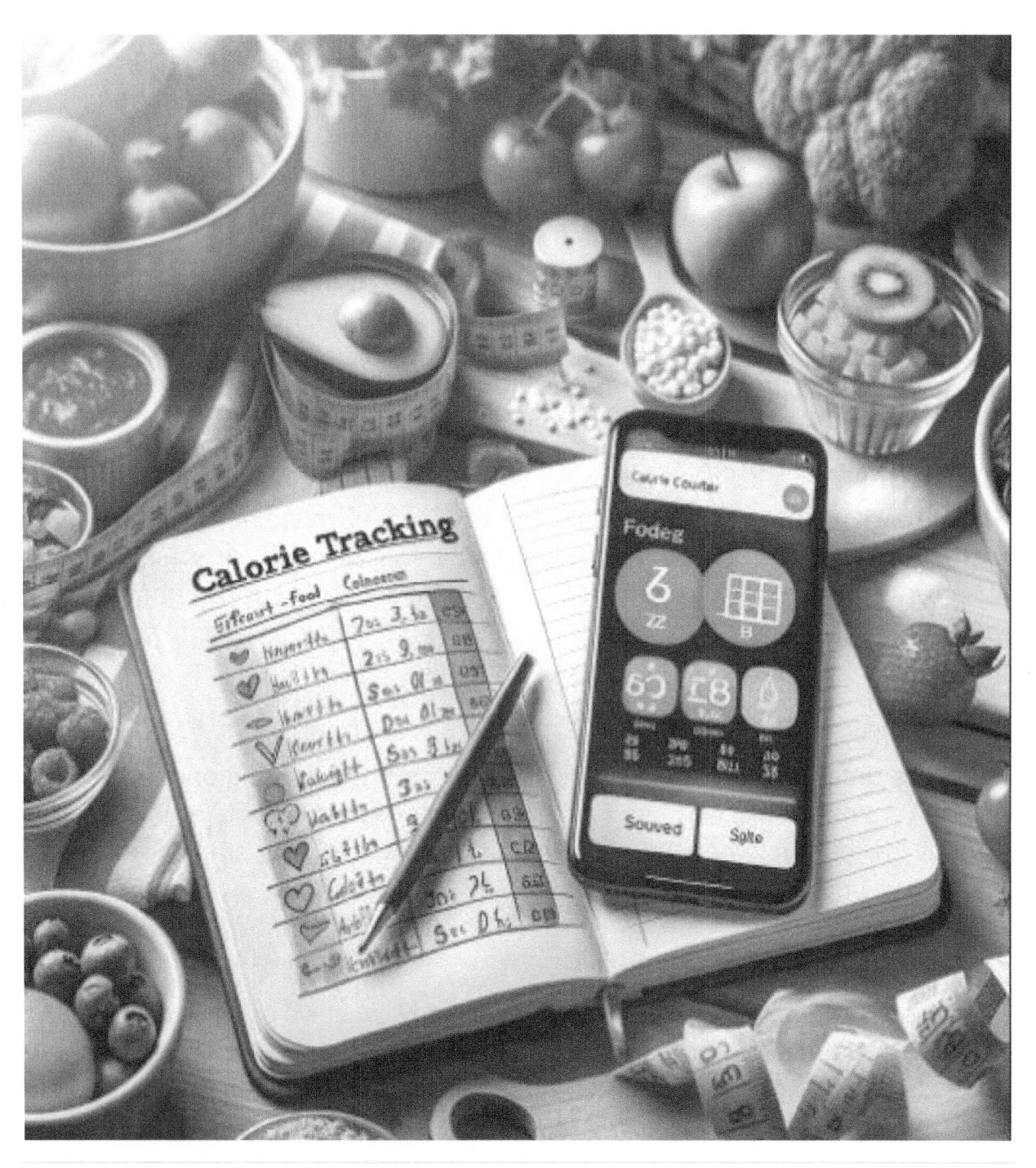

Chapter 4:
MEAL PLANNING AND CULINARY INSPIRATION

Organizing Weekly Meals for Endomorphs

It requires thoughtful planning to cater to the specific metabolic needs of individuals with an endomorph body type. Manage carbohydrate intake, increase protein intake, and include healthy fats. To help those with endomorph body types manage their diet effectively, here's a guide that simplifies these principles:

Start With Basics: If you have an endomorph body type, you naturally store energy as fat. A low-carb, high-protein, and balanced-fat diet is recommended to manage this. These principles will guide you effectively.

- **Protein is Key (Aim for a daily consume of 1g per pound of bodyweight)**

    Aim to include a lean protein source in every meal. Good options, as mentioned before, include chicken breast, turkey, lean beef, fish like salmon or trout, tofu, and eggs. Protein helps in muscle repair and maintenance and also keeps you feeling full longer.

    Visual Portion Guide: A palm-sized portion for meats, a fist-sized portion for carbs, two fist-sized portions for veggies, and a thumb-sized portion for fats.

- **Healthy Fats (Aim for a daily consume of 45-75g of fat based on your weight and gender)**

    Don't shy away from fats; just choose the right kinds, such as avocados, olive oil, nuts, seeds, and fatty fish. They contribute to satiety and provide essential fatty acids. A small portion of healthy fats should complement each meal.

- **Carbs + Veggies (Fill up your daily calories with carbs once you got the daily dose of protein and fat)**

    Opt for low-glycemic, fibrous vegetables and whole grains. Spinach, kale, broccoli, and cauliflower are great as they provide micronutrients and very low calories. Complex carbs, such as sweet potatoes, brown rice, or quinoa, should be consumed in smaller portions after workouts so they can be utilized for recovery (in the chapter before I listed the healthier options included the grams of carbs for 100g of product).

Guidelines Meal Plan

These are broad guidelines for each meal that you can follow. If you do not like having a strict plan, you can use these guidelines to make yourself a diet plan. In the next section I'm going to provide you with a more extensive and detailed list of recipes you might want to try!

Monday to Sunday Breakfast

Start your day with protein and fiber-rich options. These meals boost your metabolism without overloading on carbs. Good examples can be scrambled eggs with spinach and tomatoes, or Greek yogurt with a handful of berries - we'll see more recipes later in the chapter.

Lunches

The aim is to balance lean protein, complex carbs, and vegetables for sustained energy. Examples can be grilled chicken or fish with a quinoa salad and lots of greens, or a turkey and avocado wrap with a side salad.

Dinners

Focus on lighter carb intake. Dinner should be satisfying but not heavy. Ideally eat it two to three hours before going to sleep for optimal digestion.

Try baked salmon with steamed broccoli and a small sweet potato, or stir-fried tofu with mixed vegetables in olive oil.

Snacks (one or two per day)

Keep it protein-rich and convenient. Greek yogurt, nuts, sliced apples with almond butter, or cottage cheese with pineapple are good choices. Especially when working out, a snack can help you get enough nutrients to recover and replenish your body.

Shopping and Prep

Stick to your shopping list. Get proteins and grains in bulk at the beginning of the week. Chop vegetables and store them for easy access. Having prepared ingredients makes it easier to stick to your meal plan.

Also, do your best to diversify your protein and carb sources to ensure you receive all necessary nutrients and keep meals interesting. Different proteins provide essential amino acids, and varied carbs from whole grains and vegetables offer vitamins, minerals, and fibers for optimal digestion and daily energy.

Breakfast Recipes

Note: The guidelines suggest average portion sizes based on gender but recognize individual nutritional needs vary. This serves as a general indication suitable for most people. Also, some people might like some of these dishes as a lunch too, that's still fine!

Spinach and Feta Omelet

Ingredients :

- up to 3 eggs
- salt, pepper
- olive oil
- 30 to 50g of feta cheese.

Preparation :

- Whisk 2 or 3 eggs (for a man) and 1 or eggs (for a woman) with a dash of salt and pepper in a mixing bowl.

- Warm up 1 teaspoon of olive oil in a non-stick frying pan on medium flame. Toss in 1 cup of fresh spinach and stir-fry until it wilts slightly (it will take about 1-2 minutes).

- Next, turn down the flame, then drizzle the whisked eggs over the spinach. Wait for the edges to firm up before scattering 50g (for men) or 30g (for women) of feta cheese, crumbled, over one side of the omelet. Carefully fold the omelet over to encase the cheese.

- Continue cooking until the eggs firm up and the cheese starts to ooze a bit.

- Lastly, put it on a plate and enjoy it while it's hot.

Almond Butter Berry Smoothie

Ingredients :

- 1 and a half cups of unsweetened almond milk
- 3 tablespoons of almond butter
- 1 cup of frozen mixed berries
- 1 scoop of the protein powder
- Handful of spinach leaves

Preparation :

- Mix together 1 cup and a half of unsweetened almond milk with 3 tablespoons of almond butter, 1 cup of frozen mixed berries, a handful of spinach leaves, and 1 scoop of the protein powder (any powder works well) in a blender.

- Whizz everything on a high setting until it turns silky and lush.

- Then, pour it into a glass and drink it up, enjoying the taste!

Greek Yogurt Parfait

Ingredients:

- 20 almonds
- Chia seeds
- Fresh fruit (berries and apples are recommended)
- 1 cup (or less for women) of Greek yogurt

Preparation :

- Start with 1 cup of Greek yogurt for a man or ½ cup for a woman in a bowl or glass.

- Sprinkle in 20 almonds, add 1 tablespoon of chia seeds, and toss in a good amount of fresh berries like strawberries, blueberries, or raspberries (one apple is a good option too).

- Feel free to make another set of these layers if you're feeling fancy, and top it off with a few berries for a nice touch!

Scrambled Tofu

Ingredients:

- 100 to 200g of firm tofu
- Turmeric
- Garlic
- One onion
- Handful of spinach leaves
- Salt
- Pepper
- Avocado (optional).

Preparation :

- Take 200g (for men) or 100g (for women) of firm tofu and break it down into pieces right into a pan that's on medium heat.

- Toss in a dash of turmeric for a sunny hue, a clove of garlic all minced up, and half an onion that's been diced to add a burst of flavor.

- Stir through a cup of fresh spinach until it softens and the tofu gets nice and warm throughout. A little shake of salt and pepper can go in according to what tastes good to you.

- When it's time to serve, lay it out with half an avocado, thinly sliced, on the side.

Cottage Cheese Bowl

Ingredients:

- 1 cup of cottage chees
- One cucumber
- Handful of cherry tomatoes
- Black pepper.

Preparation :

- Take a bowl and mix in some cottage cheese. 1 cup for men and ½ cup for women.

- Throw in some diced cucumber and cherry tomatoes that you've cut in half for a bit of crunch and a burst of freshness.

- Add a sprinkle of black pepper if you like to have a tasty and nutritious breakfast!

Protein Pancakes

Ingredients:

- pancakes
- Almond flour
- A couple of eggs
- Protein powder (one scoop needed)
- Peanut butter.

Preparation :

- Start by mixing together 1 cup of almond flour, a couple of eggs (for men) or just one (for women), along with a scoop of whey protein until you've got a smooth batter.

- Get your non-stick skillet warmed up over a medium flame and then gently pour in bits of the batter to shape your pancakes.

- Wait for those little bubbles to pop up on the top, then flip them over and cook until they're a nice shade of golden.

- Lastly, slather a tablespoon of natural peanut butter on top while they're still warm.

Egg Muffins

Ingredients:

- Three to six eggs
- 100g lean turkey bacon
- Onions
- Mushrooms
- Peppers.

Preparation :

- Getting your oven warmed up to 350°F (175°C) is the first step.

- In a bowl, open 6 eggs (for men), or just 3 (for women), and give them a good whisk. Toss in your peppers, onions and mushrooms works well—to get a nice mix of different vegetables

- Then, add 100g of chopped lean turkey bacon to the bowl.

- Now, take this mixture and pour it into greased muffin tins, filling each one about three-quarters of the way.

- Put them into the oven for about 20 minutes, just until they're set!

Note: you can consider making some extra muffins and have breakfast for a few extra days!

Chia Seed Pudding

Ingredients:

- Chia seeds
- A cup of almond milk
- Strawberries (blueberries, raspberries, apples and bananas works well too)

Preparation :

- Start by tossing 3 tablespoons of chia seeds into a bowl or jar, then pour in a cup of almond milk.

- Mix them together and let the concoction chill in the fridge overnight; it'll get nice and thick.

- When you wake up, give the pudding a good stir to get that even, creamy texture, then crown it with slices of fresh strawberries or other fruits you like.

Note: fantastic breakfast to up your fiber and Omega-3 intake

Avocado Toast

Ingredients:

- Avocado
- Whole grain bread
- Egg
- Sautéed kale (optional).

Preparation :

- Take half an avocado, give it a good mash, and slather it on a slice of toast made from whole-grain bread.

- Next, gently lay a poached egg on top for that extra touch.

- Don't forget a side of sautéed kale if you like—aim for a full cup if you're a man, or half a cup if you're a woman.

Turkey Sausage and Veggie Skillet

Ingredients:

- 100 to 200g of lean turkey sausage slices
- Bell pepper (other vegetables such as carrots, tomatoes or broccoli works well too).

Preparation :

- Heat up a pan on medium, and cook some lean turkey sausage slices in it 200g for men, 100g for women - until they turn a nice shade of brown.

- Then, add in bell pepper slices for a little extra flavor and color.

Mixed Berry Oatmeal

Ingredients:

- Rolled oats
- Unsweetened almond milk (any milk you like/digest is okay)
- Cinnamon powder
- Fresh berries
- Flaxseeds (optional).

Preparation :

- Heat up half a cup of rolled oats (for men) or a third of a cup (for women), in some water or unsweetened almond milk until they're soft.

- Add just a bit of cinnamon to give it some flavor.

- Once it's done, throw on a bunch of fresh berries - blueberries, raspberries, and some sliced strawberries work great.

- For an extra crunch, add a tablespoon of flaxseeds or hemp seeds on top

Avocado and Salmon Bagel

Ingredients:

- Whole-grain bagel
- Light cheese (any type you like)
- 50f of smoked salmon
- Black pepper
- Lemon (optional).

Preparation :

- Pop a whole-grain bagel in the toaster and cut it into two halves.

- Smear a bit of light cream cheese on each piece.

- Then, lay some thinly sliced smoked salmon on one side - 50g for men, 30g for women - and some mashed avocado on the other.

- Give it a sprinkle of black pepper and a dash of lemon juice to taste nicely.

Peanut Butter Banana Smoothie

Ingredients:

- Banana
- Unsweetened almond milk (any milk you like and can digest well is okay)
- Peanut butter
- Protein powder
- Ice

Preparation :

- Throw a banana into the blender along with a cup of unsweetened almond milk, a couple of tablespoons of natural peanut butter, and a scoop of your favorite protein powder, be it vanilla or chocolate.

- Toss in some ice cubes to make the smoothie thicker.

Note; Ideal breakfast before a workout or when you need something quick to keep you going.

Veggie Breakfast Hash

Ingredients:

- Sweet potatoes
- 2 eggs
- Vegetables (red bell pepper and zucchini are recommended, others work well too)
- Olive oil
- Salt pepper
- Paprika (optional)

Preparation :

- Chop up some sweet potatoes into small pieces - for men half a cup works well (a third of cup for women)

- Get them in the oven and roast them till they're nice and soft.

- Meanwhile, in a skillet, cook up some chopped onion, red bell pepper, and zucchini with a bit of olive oil just until they start getting tender.

- Throw in those roasted sweet potatoes. Make a little space in the middle and crack in 2 eggs if you're cooking for a man, or just one for a woman, and let them cook till they're just how you like them.

- Add a little salt, pepper, and a dash of paprika to give it some extra taste.

Egg and Spinach Breakfast Wrap

Ingredients:

- 2 eggs
- Handful of spinach leaves
- Whole-grain tortilla
- Low-fat cottage cheese
- A couple of tomatoes (optional)

Preparation :

- First, whisk up 2 eggs if you're a man, or just 1 if you're a woman, and cook them until they're scrambled. Set them aside.

- Then, in that same pan, toss in a bunch of fresh spinach and cook it until it's just wilted and tender.

- Grab a whole-grain tortilla and spread a bit of low-fat cottage cheese all over it. Pile on your scrambled eggs and that wilted spinach, and then give it a good fold to make a wrap.

- Add a couple slices of tomato and a splash of hot sauce if you like.

Alternatives for Busy People

A busy schedule requires nutritious meals that can be prepared in 5 minutes or less. These recipes are designed for endomorphs.

Avocado Egg Toast

Preparation

- Toast a slice of whole-grain bread.
- Spread mashed half avocado.
- Top with slices of a hard-boiled egg. Season with salt and pepper.

Nutty Greek Yogurt Delight

Preparation

- Mix 1 cup (men) or ½ cup (women) plain Greek yogurt.
- Add a handful of walnuts or almonds and a teaspoon of honey.

Spinach Banana Protein Shake

Preparation

- Blend 1 cup almond milk, a scoop of protein powder, half a banana, and a handful of spinach.

Lunch Recipes

Note: The guidelines suggest average portion sizes based on gender but recognize individual nutritional needs vary. This serves as a general indication suitable for most people. Also, some people might like some of these dishes as a breakfast too, that's still fine!

Chicken Quinoa Salad

Ingredients:

- 150 to 200g of chicken breast
- 50 to 100g of quinoa
- Salt
- Pepper
- Oive oil
- Salad greens
- Avocado
- Cucumber
- lemon (optional)

Preparation :

- Season 200g (men) or 150g (women) chicken breast with salt, pepper, and a tiny bit of olive oil. Grill over medium heat until cooked, approximately 6-7 minutes per side. Let it rest before slicing thinly.

- As you do that, cook quinoa as per package instructions; cool slightly.

- Next, in a large bowl, toss the quinoa with mixed salad greens, half a sliced avocado, diced cucumber, and the grilled chicken slices.

- Lastly, drizzle over the salad 2 teaspoons of olive oil, fresh lemon juice to taste, salt, and pepper.

Turkey Avocado Wrap

Ingredients:

- Whole - grain wrap
- Avocado
- 70 to 100g of turkey slices
- Lettuce
- A couple of tomatoes
- Salt
- Pepper

Preparation :

- Put down a whole-grain wrap on a flat surface.

- Smear a quarter of an avocado right onto that wrap. Then, place 100g of thin turkey slices on it if you're making it for a man or 70g if it's for a woman.

- Toss on some shredded lettuce and a few tomato slices. A little bit of salt and pepper for taste, and then roll it up nice and tight so everything stays inside.

- Cut it in half and there you go, enjoy your lunch!

Beef and Broccoli Stir-Fry

Ingredients:

- 100 to 150g of lean beef
- Soy sauce
- Broccoli
- 50 to 100g of cauliflower rice.

Preparation :

- Take 150g (men) or 100g (women) of lean beef. Stir-fry the beef slices in a hot pan or wok with a tablespoon of low-sodium soy sauce until browned.

- Add broccoli and continue to cook until the vegetables are tender-crisp.

- Serve the stir-fry over a steamed cauliflower rice for a low-carb alternative to traditional rice.

Lentil Soup

Ingredients:

- 1 and a half cup of lentils
- 1 to 2 carrots
- 1 celery
- spinach leaves
- salt
- pepper other herbs (optional)
- lemon (optional)
- 2 slices of whole - grain bread (optional)50 to 100g of cauliflower rice.

Preparation :

- Rinse 1 and a half cup (men) or 1 cup (women) of lentils under cold water.

- In a large pot, bring lentils to boil in vegetable broth, then lower the heat to simmer.

- Add diced carrots, celery, and a handful of spinach leaves. Season with salt, pepper, and any herbs you like.

- Simmer until the lentils are tender, about 20-25 minutes.

- Adjust the seasoning and serve warm with a squeeze of lemon for an extra flavor - Also eat two slices of whole-grain bread if you want to

Tuna Salad Stuffed Bell Peppers

Ingredients:

- 100 to 150g of tuna
- Greek yogurt
- Salt
- 2 bell peppers
- Cucumber (optional)
- 1 slice of whole-grain bread.

Preparation :

- Mix 150g (men) or 100g (women) of tuna with 2 tablespoons of Greek yogurt, adding salt and pepper to taste.

- Cut bell peppers in half lengthwise, removing seeds and membranes.

- Spoon the tuna mixture into each bell pepper half. Serve with slices of cucumber on the side and a slice of whole-grain bread..

Note. This meal won't have as many calories as other meals. This is a light lunch that on a hot day or on a day you sit a lot aka not much movement is great!

Shrimp Avocado Salad

Ingredients:

- 100 to 150g of cooked shrimp avocado
- Cherry tomatoes
- Green salad
- Salt
- Pepper
- Olive oil.

Preparation :

- Throw together 150g of cooked shrimp for men, or 100g for women, with half an avocado sliced up, a good bunch of mixed salad greens, and some cherry tomatoes cut in half.

- Mix up some lime juice, a couple of teaspoons of olive oil, and a pinch each of salt and pepper for the dressing.

- Pour this zesty lime vinaigrette over your salad, give it a light toss to make sure everything gets a nice coating, and then it's ready to serve.

Grilled Salmon and Asparagus

Ingredients:

- 150 to 200g of salmon
- 80 to 100g of quinoa (optional)
- Salt
- Pepper
- Lemon.

Preparation :

- Sprinkle a bit of salt, pepper, and a bit of lemon juice over a salmon fillet—2000g for men, 150g for women.

- Pop the salmon and some asparagus spears on the grill. Cook them until the salmon is right, kind of opaque and flaky when you poke it with a fork, and the asparagus has that perfect crunch.

- Serve it with some cooked quinoa beside it for a meal, if you like

Sweet Potato and Black Bean Bowl

Ingredients:

- 100 to 150g of sweet potatoes
- ½ cup of black beans
- Red bell pepper
- A couple of green onions
- Handful of corn kernels
- Olive oil
- Sumin
- Salt
- Pepper.

Preparation :

- Roast cubed sweet potatoes (150g for men, 100g for women) in the oven at 400°F until tender and slightly caramelized, about 25-30 minutes.

- In a bowl, mix the roasted sweet potatoes with cooked black beans (½ cup for men, ⅓ cup for women), a handful of fresh corn kernels, diced red bell pepper, and sliced green onions.

- For dressing, whisk together lime juice, a teaspoon of olive oil, cumin, salt, and pepper. Drizzle over the bowl and toss to combine.

Mushroom and Spinach Frittata

Ingredients:

- 2 to 4 eggs
- 1 cup of sliced mushrooms
- 1 cup of spinach
- milk
- salt
- pepper
- olive oil

Preparation :

- Whisk together 4 eggs (men) or 2 eggs (women) with a splash of milk, salt, and pepper.

- Sauté sliced mushrooms (1 cup) and spinach (1 cup) in a skillet with a teaspoon of olive oil until the spinach is wilted and the mushrooms are golden.

- Pour the egg mixture over the vegetables. Cook over low heat until the edges start to set, then transfer to a 350°F oven to finish cooking, about 10-15 minutes.

- Serve warm, sliced into wedges.

Quinoa and Vegetable Stuffed Peppers

Ingredients:

- ½ cup of quinoa
- A couple of bell peppers
- Zucchini
- A few cherry tomatoes
- Chopped spinach
- Garlic powder
- Oregano
- Salt
- Pepper
- Feta cheese (optional).

Preparation :

- Cook quinoa according to package instructions. Halve bell peppers lengthwise and remove seeds. In a mixing bowl, combine the cooked quinoa (½ cup for men, ⅓ cup for women) with diced zucchini, cherry tomatoes, and chopped spinach. Season with garlic powder, oregano, salt, and pepper.

- Stuff the mixture into the bell pepper halves.

- Bake at 375°F for about 20 minutes.

- Top with a sprinkle of feta cheese just before serving.

Chickpea Salad Sandwich

Ingredients:

- two slices of whole-grain bread (ideally whole-grain)
- ½ cup of chickpeas
- celery
- red onion
- handful parsley
- cup of Greek yogurt
- salt
- pepper

Preparation :

- Mash 1(2 cup of cooked chickpeas in a bowl. Mix in diced celery, red onion, and a small handful of chopped fresh parsley.

- Stir in a tablespoon of Greek yogurt and a squeeze of lemon juice for creaminess and flavor. Season with salt and pepper.

- Spread the chickpea salad on whole-grain bread and add lettuce leaves for crunch.

Asian Chicken Lettuce Wraps

Ingredients:

- 150 to 200g of ground chicken
- Carrots
- onion
- soy sauce
- sesame oil
- honey and garlic
- lettuce leaves (optional)
- 1 slice of whole-grain

Preparation :

- Cook ground chicken (200g for men, 150g for women) in a pan, breaking it apart with a spoon.

- Once cooked, add finely chopped water chestnuts, shredded carrots, and diced onions.

- For the sauce, mix soy sauce, sesame oil, a touch of honey, and minced garlic.

- Toss the chicken mixture in the sauce and cook until everything is well-coated. Spoon the mixture into lettuce leaves and serve. Add a slice of whole-grain bread to get some carbs in.

Alternatives for Busy People

A busy schedule requires nutritious meals that can be prepared in 5 minutes or less. These recipes are designed for endomorphs.

Tuna in Lettuce Cups

Preparation

- Combine a can of drained tuna with Greek yogurt, lemon juice, and seasonings.
- Spoon the mixture into romaine lettuce leaves. Add diced veggies like cucumbers or tomatoes if you like.

Chickpea Veggie Toss

Preparation

- Mix canned chickpeas (rinsed and drained) with halved cherry tomatoes, diced cucumber, and arugula leaves.
- Dress with olive oil, lemon juice, and season with salt and pepper.
- Eat also a sliced of whole-grain bread (optional but recommended)

Cheese and Turkey Pinwheels

Preparation

- Spread a layer of cream cheese (optional) on turkey slices, add a slice of cheese, and roll up.
- Secure with toothpicks and pair with baby carrots for crunch.

Dinner Recipes

Note: The guidelines suggest average portion sizes based on gender but recognize individual nutritional needs vary. This serves as a general indication suitable for most people.

Baked Cod with Roasted Veggies

Ingredients:

- 175 to 225g of cod fillet
- lemon slices
- salt
- pepper
- olive oil
- lemon (optional)

Preparation :

- Preheat your oven to 375°F (190°C). Place 175g to 225g of cod fillet on a baking sheet.

- Season with lemon slices, dried herbs, salt, and pepper. Surround with Brussels sprouts and carrot chunks tossed in 1 tbsp olive oil.

- Bake for 20-25 minutes until the fish flakes easily and vegetables are tender.

- Drizzle lemon juice over the cod before serving for an extra flavour.

Zucchini Noodles with Turkey Meatballs

Ingredients:

- 150g to 200g of meatballs
- 2 medium zucchini (for the noodles) minced garlic
- Salt
- Pepper
- Parsley
- 1 egg

Preparation :

- For the meatballs, mix 200g (men) or 150g (women) ground turkey with minced garlic, chopped parsley, salt, pepper, and 1 beaten egg for binding.

- Form into small balls and bake on a lined tray at 375°F (190°C) for 20 minutes.

- Spiralize 2 medium zucchinis for the noodles. Sauté zoodles in a pan with a touch of olive oil for 2-3 minutes.

- Serve the meatballs over zoodles with a hearty spoonful of marinara sauce.

Stuffed Acorn Squash

Ingredients:

- 100 to 150g of ground turkey
- minced garlic
- onion
- ½ cup of cooked quinoa
- A corn squash
- Seeds
- Olive oil
- Dried cranberries
- Handful of fresh spinach leaves

Preparation :

- Cut an acorn squash in half and scoop out the seeds. Brush with olive oil and season.

- Roast cut-side down at 400°F (200°C) for about 25 minutes.

- Meanwhile, cook 150g (men) or 100g (women) ground turkey with minced garlic, onion, and spices until browned.

- Mix in ½ cup cooked quinoa, a handful of dried cranberries, and chopped spinach.

- Stuff the mixture into the roasted squash halves and bake for another 15 minutes.

Grilled Chicken and Vegetable Kebabs

Ingredients:

- 150 to 200g of chicken breast
- A couple of zucchini
- Two bell peppers
- Pepper
- Other herbs (optional).
- Onion
- Greek yogurt
- One cucumber
- Salt

Preparation :

- Cut 200g (men) or 150g (women) of chicken breast into chunks.

- Thread onto skewers alternately with chunks of bell peppers, zucchini, and onion.

- Brush lightly with olive oil; season with salt, pepper, and your choice of herbs.

- Grill on medium heat, turning occasionally, until chicken is cooked through.

- Serve with a side of Greek yogurt mixed with cucumber and dill as a dip.

Beef Stew

Ingredients:

- 150 to 200g of lean beef
- 30 to 50g of tomatoes
- Pepper
- 2 carrots
- Celery
- A couple of onions
- Calt
- Thyme (optional) and bay leaves (optional).

Preparation :

- In a large pot, brown 200g (men) or 150g (women) lean beef chunks in a bit of olive oil. Add chopped tomatoes, diced carrots, celery, and onions.

- Cover with beef broth and bring to a boil. Simmer on low heat for 1-2 hours until the beef is tender.

- Season with thyme, bay leaves, salt, and pepper for depth of flavor.

Cauliflower Crust Pizza

Ingredients:

- Premade cauliflower crust
- Egg
- Salt
- 90 to 130g of shredded mozzarella
- Vegetables (carrots, zucchini and broccoli works well, but choose any you like)

Preparation :

- Use a pre-made cauliflower crust or make your own by processing cauliflower in a food processor, then steaming and squeezing out the moisture.

- Mix with an egg, salt, and spices, then spread into a thin circle on a baking sheet. Pre-bake at 400°F (200°C) for 15-20 minutes.

- Add tomato sauce, 130g (men) or 90g (women) shredded mozzarella, and your favorite vegetable toppings. Bake for another 10 minutes until the cheese is bubbly.

Spaghetti Squash Bolognese

Ingredients:

- Spaghetti squash
- Lean ground beef (200g for men, 150g for women)
- garlic
- Onion
- Tomato sauce

Preparation :

- Halve a spaghetti squash and scoop out seeds. Roast cut-side down at 400°F (200°C) for 40 minutes.

- Meanwhile, cook 200g (men) or 150g (women) lean ground beef with garlic, onion, and tomato sauce.

- Scrape the roasted squash with a fork to create "spaghetti," then top with the meat sauce.

Pork Tenderloin with Green Beans

Ingredients:

- 150 to 200g of pork tenderloin
- Salt
- Pepper
- herbs (optional)
- handful of green beans
- small sweet potato
- vegetables you like (cucumber, carrots, tomatoes, zucchini…)

Preparation :

- Season a 200g (men) or 150g (women) pork tenderloin with salt, pepper, and herbs. Roast at 375°F (190°C) for 25-30 minutes.

- Steam green beans and bake a small sweet potato as a side.

- Slice the tenderloin and serve with vegetables.

Chicken Fajita Bowl

Ingredients:

- 150 to 200g of chicken breast
- Bell peppers
- Onion
- Avocado
- Fajita seasonings

Preparation :

- Slice 150 to 200g of chicken breast, bell peppers, and onions.

- Sauté in a pan with fajita seasoning until cooked.

- Serve the mixture over a bed of lettuce topped

Salmon Patty Burgers

Ingredients:

- 200g of canned salmon
- Egg
- A couple of onions
- Salt
- Pepper
- A couple of lettuce leaves

Preparation :

- Mix 200g (men) or 150g (women) canned salmon with an egg, chopped onions, salt, and pepper. Form into patties and grill until cooked through.

- Serve on lettuce leaves as "buns" with a side of roasted sweet.

Garlic Herb Roasted Chicken and Root Vegetables

Ingredients:

- 200g of chicken drumsticks
- crushed garlic
- olive oil
- rosemary
- thyme
- two carrots
- 50 to 100g of sweet potatoes

Preparation :

- Marinate 200g of chicken drumsticks in a mix of crushed garlic, olive oil, rosemary, and thyme.

- Arrange on a baking tray with cubed beets, carrots, and 50 to 100g of sweet potatoes, all lightly tossed in olive oil and seasoning.

- Roast at 425°F (220°C) for about 40 minutes, turning halfway through, until the chicken is fully cooked and vegetables are fork-tender.

Baked Lemon Pepper Fish with Green Beans

Ingredients:

- 200g fo fillets
- lemon slices
- ½ cup of green beans

Preparation :

- Season tilapia fillets (200g for men, 150g for women) with lemon pepper seasoning and a drizzle of lemon juice.

- Lay on a lightly greased baking dish along with green beans.

- Add a few lemon slices on top for extra flavor and bake at 375°F (190°C) for 15-20 minutes, until the fish is opaque and flakes easily.

Coconut Curry Vegetable Lentil Stew

Ingredients:

- 50g of sweet potatoes
- one bell pepper
- cup of lentils
- onions
- minced ginger
- garlic
- coconut oil
- curry powder

Preparation :

- In a large pot, sauté a base of onions, minced ginger, and garlic in coconut oil. Add a tablespoon of curry powder or to taste, stirring until fragrant. Mix in 50g of diced sweet potatoes, a bell pepper, and a cup of lentils, covering with coconut milk and vegetable stock.

- Simmer until the lentils are tender and the vegetables are cooked through, about 25/30 minutes.

Spicy Ground Turkey and Quinoa Stuffed Peppers

Ingredients:

- 100g of quinoa
- 150 to 200g of ground turkey
- Onion
- 2 bell peppers
- minced garlic
- cumin powder
- chili powder
- corn
- shredded cheese (optional)

Preparation :

- Hollow out bell peppers and set aside. Cook 50 to 100g of quinoa as directed.

- Sauté ground turkey (200g for men, 150g for women) with onion, minced garlic, cumin, and chili powder until browned.

- Mix the turkey with the cooked quinoa and corn.

- Stuff the mixture into the bell peppers, bake in a preheated oven at 350°F (175°C) for 25 minutes.

- A sprinkle of shredded cheese in the last few minutes of baking adds a tasty finish.

Greek Chickpea and Vegetable Salad

Ingredients:

- 1 cup of chickpeas
- diced cucumber
- red onion slices
- two diced bell peppers
- olive oil
- minced garlic
- oregano
- salt and pepper
- 1 to 2 slices of whole-grain bread
- feta cheese (optional)

Preparation :

- Toss together chickpeas (1 cup for men, ½ cup for women), diced cucumber, cherry tomatoes, red onion slices, and diced bell pepper. Add olives and crumbled feta cheese to taste.

- Dress with a vinaigrette of olive oil, minced garlic, oregano, salt, and pepper. Also eat 1 to 2 slices of whole-grain bread.

Alternatives for Busy People

A busy schedule requires nutritious meals that can be prepared in 5 minutes or less. These recipes are designed for endomorphs.

Salmon Quick Fix

Preparation :

- Season a salmon fillet with lemon, dill, and seasonings. Place in a microwave-safe dish and cover.

- Microwave on high for 3-4 minutes. Serve with quick microwave-steamed broccoli.

Beef Spinach Sauté

Preparation :

- Warm pre-cooked beef slices in a pan, toss in a handful of spinach until just wilted.

- Flavor with a splash of soy sauce and sesame seeds. Add a slice or two of rye bread (optional)

Scrambled Egg & Avocado Plate

Preparation :

- Quickly scramble 2 eggs. Serve over fresh spinach with avocado slices.

- A sprinkle of hot sauce adds flavor without extra calories.

Healthy Snacks and Sides Recipes

I would consider adding a snack to your daily meals when you do the intense training session to make sure your body recovers well and/or is full of energy for the upcoming session! On days where you simply go for long walks or stretch, I would avoid this or suggest cutting the portion in half.

Here are five valuable options:

Greek Yogurt with Berries

A cup of plain Greek yogurt mixed with a variety of berries (strawberries, blueberries, raspberries) offers a high-protein snack with the added benefits of antioxidants and fiber. The probiotics in yogurt are great for digestive health, while the natural sweetness of berries satisfies sugar cravings without the guilt.

Hummus and Veggie Sticks

Combining a rich, creamy hummus with crunchy vegetables like carrots, cucumbers, and bell peppers provides a satisfying snack that's rich in protein and fiber. This combination keeps you full for longer periods, aiding in weight management and providing essential nutrients.

Almond Butter and Apple Slices

A small serving of almond butter with crisp apple slices makes for a delicious snack that balances sweetness with healthy fats and protein. The fiber in the apple and the monounsaturated fats in the almond butter can help stabilize blood sugar levels.

Quinoa Salad

A small bowl of quinoa salad with mixed vegetables (tomatoes, cucumbers, spinach) and a lemon vinaigrette offers a light yet nutritious side dish, rich in protein and all nine essential amino acids. It's a gluten-free option that also provides a good dose of fiber and iron.

Roasted Chickpeas

Seasoned and roasted until crispy, chickpeas make an excellent snack or side dish. They're a fantastic source of protein, fiber, and can be flavored in numerous ways (spicy, savory, or even slightly sweet), making them a versatile option to keep snacking interesting.

Dining out and social eating

When it comes to dining out or engaging in social eating, the key is preparation and mindset. Here are practical and mindset tips, supported by real-life examples:

Preview the Menu : Before heading out, check the restaurant's menu online. Look for dishes that fit within your dietary goals. For example, opting for grilled over fried foods or selecting sides of vegetables instead of high-carb options like fries or mashed potatoes.

Don't Hesitate to Customize : Don't be shy about asking for modifications to your meal. For instance, substituting salad for a side of fries or requesting the dressing on the side. A real-life example includes someone requesting a lettuce wrap instead of a bun for their burger, aligning the meal more closely with their dietary needs.

Practice Portion Control : When portions are large, consider sharing a dish with a friend or packing half of it to take home. This approach allows you to enjoy your meal without overindulging.

Mindful Eating : Focus on your meal and enjoy each bite, which can help prevent overeating. A practical tip is to put your utensil down between bites, encouraging slower eating and better digestion.

Navigate Social Pressure : Sometimes, social situations can lead to pressure to eat outside of your preferences. Politely declining or suggesting alternative options, like meeting at a café that offers healthier choices, can help you maintain your dietary goals without isolating yourself socially.

Remember, the goal of dining out or social eating is to enjoy the experience with your friends or family. Balancing enjoyment with mindful choices allows you to maintain your dietary goals without feeling deprived.

Chapter 5:
A 28-DAY NUTRITIONAL PLAN FOR ENDOMORPHS

5 Nutritional Notes to Keep in Mind

- In this plan I put all healthy options for breakfast, lunch and dinner to make sure you have precise guidelines. However, **it is still acceptable to eat some "not super healthy" food once a week**. Out of 21 weekly meals, if 1 is not healthy, it will not hinder your progress - Just consume it in moderation avoiding big portions

- I've taken the time to **estimate the calories for each meal, aiming to give you a comprehensive overview**. On average, a woman consumes about 1,400 to 1,600 calories daily, while a man consumes around 2,200 to 2,600 calories (or even more). Remember, these figures include the three main meals. Plus, you should consider adding a snack of your choice (or even two a day) - I've suggested some healthy options in the previous chapter in the section *"Healthy Snacks and Side Recipes"*.

- Note that the **calories mentioned per food are a rough estimate**. It can vary based on the amount of vegetables or toppings you put other than the main ingredient. If you're not used to counting calories, don't go crazy counting them every single meal.

- It's important to note that **your caloric needs could vary.** Factors such as your age, height, and daily activity levels play a crucial role in determining this. So, feel free to adjust the portions slightly to better suit your individual needs.

- **For weight management**: to lose weight, consume 300 to 500 calories less than you burn daily. If gaining weight is your goal (I don't think it is but many a small percentage of you would like to know this), aim for a surplus of 300 to 500 calories. This principle must be the foundation of your weight loss journey.

Week 1 Plan

Day 1:

Breakfast : Spinach and Feta Omelet

- Men : 2 or 3 eggs, 50g feta ≅ 450 Calories

- Women : 1 or 2 eggs, 30g feta ≅ 370 Calories

Lunch : Chicken Quinoa Salad

- Men : 200g chicken, 100g quinoa ≅ 680 Calories

- Women : 150g chicken, 50g quinoa ≅ 490 Calories

Dinner : Baked Cod with Roasted Veggies

- Men : 225g cod, 1 cup veggies ≅ 500 Calories

- Women : 175g cod, ½ cup veggies ≅ 400 Calories

Day 2:

Breakfast : Almond Butter Berry Smoothie

- Men : 3 tbsp almond butter, 1 cup berries ≅ 420 Calories

- Women : 1 to 2 tbsp almond butter, ½ cup berries ≅ 310 Calories

Lunch : Turkey Avocado Wrap

- Men : 100g turkey, ¼ avocado ≅ 620 Calories

- Women : 70g turkey, ⅛ avocado ≅ 450 Calories

Dinner : Zucchini Noodles with Turkey Meatballs

- Men : 200g meatballs ≅ 550 Calories

- Women : 150g meatballs ≅ 450 Calories

Day 3:

Breakfast : Greek Yogurt Parfait

- Men : 1 cup yogurt, almonds, fruit ≅ 410-500 Calories *(Calories are on the lower end with just berries and on the higher end if an apple is included)*
- Women : ½ cup yogurt, almonds ≅ 300-350 Calories *(Calories are on the lower end with just berries and on the higher end if an apple is included)*

Lunch : Lentil Soup

- Men : 1 and a half cup lentils ≅ 450 Calories (*Included two slices of whole-grain bread*)
- Women : 1 cup (or less) lentils ≅ 320 Calories (*Included two slices of whole-grain bread*)

Dinner : Grilled Chicken and Vegetable Kebabs

- Men : 200g chicken ≅ 460 Calories
- Women : 150g chicken ≅ 380 Calories

Day 4:

Breakfast: Scrambled Tofu

- Men : 200g tofu ≅ 300 Calories
- Women : 100g tofu ≅ 150 Calories

Lunch : Tuna Salad Stuffed Bell Peppers

- Men : 150g tuna ≅ 410 Calories
- Women : 100g tuna ≅ 330 Calories

Dinner : Beef Stew

- Men : 200g beef ≅ 530 Calories
- Women : 150g beef ≅ 400 Calories

Day 5:

Breakfast : Cottage Cheese Bowl

- Men : 1 cup cottage cheese ≅ 280 Calories
- Women : ½ cup cottage cheese ≅ 140 Calories

Lunch : Beef and Broccoli Stir-Fry

- Men : 150g beef, 1 cup broccoli ≅ 450 Calories
- Women : 100g beef, ½ cup broccoli ≅ 380 Calories

Dinner : Cauliflower Crust Pizza

- Men : Cauliflower crust, 130g mozzarella ≅ 530 Calories
- Women : Cauliflower crust, 90g mozzarella ≅ 390 Calories

Day 6:

Breakfast : Protein Pancakes

- Men : 2 pancakes ≅ 350 Calories
- Women : 1 pancake ≅ 190 Calories

Lunch : Shrimp Avocado Salad

- Men : 150g shrimp ≅ 440 Calories
- Women : 100g shrimp ≅ 370 Calories

Dinner : Spaghetti Squash Bolognese

- Men : 200g ground beef ≅ 550 Calories
- Women : 150g ground beef ≅ 410 Calories

Day 7:

Breakfast : Egg Muffins

- Men : 6 eggs (3 muffins) ≅ 500 Calories

- Women : 3 eggs (1-2 muffins) ≅ 250 Calories

Lunch : Grilled Salmon and Asparagus

- Men : 200g salmon ≅ 450 Calories (considering 100g of quinoa too)

- Women : 150g salmon ≅ 370 Calories (considering 80g of quinoa too)

Dinner : Chicken Fajita Bowl

- Men : 200g chicken ≅ 490 Calories

- Women : 150g chicken ≅ 380 Calories

Week 2 Plan

Day 8:

Breakfast : Chia Seed Pudding

- Men : 3 tbsp chia seeds, 1 cup almond milk ≅ 380-450 Calories *(based on the fruit you choose to add)*

- Women : 2 tbsp chia seeds, ¾ cup almond milk ≅ 300-380 Calories *(based on the fruit you choose to add)*

Lunch : Chicken Caesar Salad

- Men : 150g chicken, 1 cup lettuce ≅ 480 Calories

- Women : 100g chicken, 1 cup lettuce ≅ 370 Calories

Dinner : Pork Tenderloin with Green Beans

- Men : 200g pork, 1 cup green beans ≅ 460 Calories

- Women : 150g pork, ½ cup green beans ≅ 390 Calories

Day 9:

Breakfast : Avocado Toast

- Men : 1 slice whole grain bread, ½ avocado ≅ 350 Calories
- Women : 1 slice whole grain bread, ¼ avocado ≅ 270 Calories

Lunch : Vegetable and Hummus Plate

- Men : ¼ cup hummus, 1 cup raw veggies ≅ 170 Calories
- Women : 2 tbsp hummus, 1 cup raw veggies ≅ 120 Calories

Dinner : Salmon Patty Burgers

- Men : 200g salmon ≅ 490 Calories
- Women : 150g salmon ≅ 380 Calories

Day 10:

Breakfast : Turkey Sausage and Veggie Skillet

- Men : 200g turkey sausage ≅ 420 Calories
- Women : 150g turkey sausage ≅ 350 Calories

Lunch : Egg Salad on Rye

- Men : 2 eggs, 2 slices rye bread ≅ 420 Calories
- Women : 1 egg, 1 slice rye bread ≅ 335 Calories

Dinner : Garlic Herb Roasted Chicken and Root Vegetables

- Men : 200g chicken, 1 cup veggies ≅ 520 Calories
- Women : 150g chicken, ½ cup veggies ≅ 430 Calories

Day 11:

Breakfast : Mixed Berry Oatmeal

- Men : ½ cup oats ≅ 310 Calories

- Women : ⅓ cup oats ≅ 230 Calories

Lunch : Quinoa and Vegetable Stuffed Peppers

- Men : ½ cup quinoa ≅ 319 Calories

- Women : ⅓ cup quinoa ≅ 213 Calories

Dinner : Baked Lemon Pepper Fish with Green Beans

- Men : 200g fish ≅ 360 Calories

- Women : 150g fish ≅ 270 Calories

Day 12:

Breakfast : Avocado and Salmon Bagel

- Men : 1 whole-grain bagel, 50g salmon ≅ 410 Calories

- Women : 1 whole-grain bagel, 30g salmon ≅ 330 Calories

Lunch : Mushroom and Spinach Frittata

- Men : 4 eggs ≅ 400 Calories

- Women : 2 eggs ≅ 200 Calories

Dinner : Beef Spinach Sauté (Quick Fix Dinner)

- Men : 200g beef, 1 cup spinach, 2 slices of rye bread ≅ 500 Calories

- Women : 150g beef, 1 cup spinach, 1 slice of rye bread ≅ 410 Calories

Day 13:

Breakfast : Veggie Breakfast Hash

- Men : ½ cup sweet potatoes ≅ 360 Calories
- Women : ⅓ cup sweet potatoes ≅ 230 Calories

Lunch : Chickpea Salad Sandwich

- Men : 1 cup chickpeas ≅ 460 Calories
- Women : ½ cup chickpeas ≅ 240 Calories

Dinner : Coconut Curry Vegetable Lentil Stew

- Men : 1 cup lentils ≅ 600 Calories
- Women : ½ cup lentils ≅ 340 Calories

Day 14:

Breakfast : Peanut Butter Banana Smoothie

- Men : 2 tbsp peanut butter ≅ 330 Calories
- Women : 1 tbsp peanut butter ≅ 250 Calories

Lunch : Asian Chicken Lettuce Wraps

- Men : 200g chicken ≅ 440 Calories
- Women : 150g chicken ≅ 310 Calories

Dinner : Greek Chickpea and Vegetable Salad

- Men : 1 cup chickpeas, veggies, 2 slices of whole-grain bread ≅ 450 Calories
- Women : ½ cup (or more) of chickpeas, veggies, 1 slices of whole-grain bread ≅ 310 Calories

Week 3 Plan

Day 15:

Breakfast : Egg and Spinach Breakfast Wrap

- Men : 2 eggs, 1 whole-grain tortilla ≅ 360 Calories

- Women : 1 egg, 1 whole-grain tortilla ≅ 270 Calories

Lunch : Sweet Potato and Black Bean Bowl

- Men : 150g sweet potatoes, ½ cup black beans ≅ 410 Calories

- Women : 100g sweet potatoes, ⅓ cup black beans ≅ 300 Calories

Dinner : Spicy Ground Turkey and Quinoa Stuffed Peppers

- Men : 200g turkey, ½ cup quinoa ≅ 550 Calories

- Women : 150g turkey, ⅓ cup quinoa ≅ 430 Calories

Day 16:

Breakfast : Avocado Egg Toast (Quick Fix Breakfast)

- Men : 1 slice whole-grain bread, ½ avocado, 1 egg ≅ 330 Calories

- Women : 1 slice whole-grain bread, ¼ avocado, 1 egg ≅ 290 Calories

Lunch : Quinoa and Vegetable Stuffed Peppers

- Men : ½ cup quinoa ≅ 320 Calories

- Women : ⅓ cup quinoa ≅ 225 Calories

Dinner : Cauliflower Crust Pizza

- Men : Cauliflower crust, 130g mozzarella ≅ 530 Calories

- Women : Cauliflower crust, 90g mozzarella ≅ 390 Calories

Day 17:

Breakfast : Mixed Berry Oatmeal

- Men : ½ cup oats ≅ 310 Calories

- Women : ⅓ cup oats ≅ 230 Calories

Lunch : Mushroom and Spinach Frittata

- Men : 4 eggs ≅ 400 Calories

- Women : 2 eggs ≅ 200 Calories

Dinner : Baked Lemon Pepper Fish with Green Beans

- Men : 200g fish ≅ 360 Calories

- Women : 150g fish ≅ 270 Calories

Day 18:

Breakfast : Peanut Butter Banana Smoothie

- Men : 2 tbsp peanut butter ≅ 330 Calories

- Women : 1 tbsp peanut butter ≅ 235 Calories

Lunch : Asian Chicken Lettuce Wraps

- Men : 200g chicken ≅ 440 Calories

- Women : 150g chicken ≅ 310 Calories

Dinner : Greek Chickpea and Vegetable Salad

- Men : 1 cup chickpeas, veggies, 2 slices of whole-grain bread ≅ 450 Calories

- Women : ½ cup (or more) of chickpeas, veggies, 1 slices of whole-grain bread ≅ 310 Calories

Day 19:

Breakfast : Cottage Cheese Bowl

- Men : 1 cup cottage cheese ≅ 220 Calories
- Women : ½ cup cottage cheese ≅ 130 Calories

Lunch : Beef and Broccoli Stir-Fry

- Men : 150g beef, 1 cup broccoli ≅ 420 Calories
- Women : 100g beef, ½ cup broccoli ≅ 340 Calories

Dinner : Spaghetti Squash Bolognese

- Men : 200g ground beef ≅ 510 Calories
- Women : 150g ground beef ≅ 390 Calories

Day 20:

Breakfast : Chia Seed Pudding

- Men : 3 tbsp chia seeds, 1 cup almond milk ≅ 380-450 Calories *(based on the fruit you choose to add)*
- Women : 2 tbsp chia seeds, ¾ cup almond milk ≅ 300-380 Calories *(based on the fruit you choose to add)*

Lunch : Tuna Salad Stuffed Bell Peppers

- Men : 150g tuna ≅ 410 Calories
- Women : 100g tuna ≅ 330 Calories

Dinner : Grilled Salmon and Asparagus

- Men : 150g salmon ≅ 350 Calories
- Women : 100g salmon ≅ 240 Calories

Day 21:

Breakfast : Scrambled Tofu

- Men : 200g tofu ≅ 230 Calories

- Women : 100g tofu ≅ 115 Calories

Lunch : Turkey Avocado Wrap

- Men : 100g turkey, ¼ avocado ≅ 590 Calories

- Women : 70g turkey, ⅛ avocado ≅ 390 Calories

Dinner : Zucchini Noodles with Turkey Meatballs

- Men : 200g meatballs ≅ 510 Calories

- Women : 150g meatballs ≅ 410 Calories

Week 4 Plan

Day 22:

Breakfast : Mixed Berry Oatmeal

- Men : ½ cup oats, 1 cup berries ≅ 380 Calories

- Women : ⅓ cup oats, ½ cup berries ≅ 300 Calories

Lunch : Vegetable and Hummus Plate

- Men : ¼ cup hummus, 1 cup raw veggies ≅ 200 Calories

- Women : 2 tbsp hummus, 1 cup raw veggies ≅ 170 Calories

Dinner : Pork Tenderloin with Green Beans

- Men : 200g pork, 1 cup green beans ≅ 500 Calories

- Women : 150g pork, ½ cup green beans ≅ 400 Calories

Day 23:

Breakfast : Avocado and Salmon Bagel

- Men : Whole grain bagel, 50g salmon, ½ avocado ≅ 430 Calories
- Women : Whole grain bagel, 30g salmon, ¼ avocado ≅ 350 Calories

Lunch : Quinoa and Vegetable Stuffed Peppers

- Men : ½ cup quinoa, 2 bell peppers ≅ 350 Calories
- Women : ⅓ cup quinoa, 2 bell peppers ≅ 240 Calories

Dinner : Baked Lemon Pepper Fish with Green Beans

- Men : 200g fish, 1 cup green beans ≅ 390 Calories
- Women : 150g fish, ½ cup green beans ≅ 300 Calories

Day 24:

Breakfast : Veggie Breakfast Hash

- Men : ½ cup sweet potatoes, 2 eggs ≅ 350 Calories
- Women : ⅓ cup sweet potatoes, 1 egg ≅ 290 Calories

Lunch : Mushroom and Spinach Frittata

- Men : 4 eggs, 1 cup spinach ≅ 420 Calories
- Women : 2 eggs, 1 cup spinach ≅ 290 Calories

Dinner : Beef Spinach Sauté (Quick Fix Dinner)

- Men : 200g beef, 1 cup spinach, 2 slices of rye bread ≅ 500 Calories
- Women : 150g beef, 1 cup spinach, 1 slice of rye bread ≅ 410 Calories

Day 25:

Breakfast : Peanut Butter Banana Smoothie

- Men : 2 tbsp peanut butter, 1 banana ≅ 350 Calories
- Women : 1 tbsp peanut butter, 1 banana ≅ 260 Calories

Lunch : Asian Chicken Lettuce Wraps

- Men : 200g chicken ≅ 440 Calories
- Women : 150g chicken ≅ 310 Calories

Dinner : Greek Chickpea and Vegetable Salad

- Men : 1 cup chickpeas, veggies, 2 slices of whole-grain bread ≅ 450 Calories
- Women : ½ cup (or more) of chickpeas, veggies, 1 slices of whole-grain bread ≅ 310 Calories

Day 26:

Breakfast : Egg and Spinach Breakfast Wrap

- Men : 2 eggs, 1 whole-grain tortilla ≅ 380 Calories
- Women : 1 egg, 1 whole-grain tortilla ≅ 280 Calories

Lunch : Sweet Potato and Black Bean Bowl

- Men : 150g sweet potatoes, ½ cup black beans ≅ 470 Calories
- Women : 100g sweet potatoes, ⅓ cup black beans ≅ 390 Calories

Dinner : Spicy Ground Turkey and Quinoa Stuffed Peppers

- Men : 200g turkey, ½ cup quinoa ≅ 560 Calories
- Women : 150g turkey, ⅓ cup quinoa ≅ 420 Calories

Day 27:

Breakfast : Avocado Egg Toast (Quick Breakfast)

- Men : 1 slice whole-grain bread, ½ avocado, 2 eggs ≅ 450 Calories
- Women : 1 slice whole-grain bread, ¼ avocado, 1 egg ≅ 360 Calories

Lunch : Chickpea Veggie Toss (Quick Lunch)

- Men : 1 cup chickpeas (+ 2 slices of whole-grain bread) ≅ 480 Calories
- Women : ½ cup chickpeas (+ 1 slice of whole-grain bread) ≅ 300 Calories

Dinner : Cauliflower Crust Pizza

- Men : Cauliflower crust, 130g mozzarella ≅ 530 Calories
- Women : Cauliflower crust, 90g mozzarella ≅ 390 Calories

Day 28:

Breakfast : Chia Seed Pudding

- Men : 3 tbsp chia seeds, 1 cup almond milk ≅ 380-450 Calories *(based on the fruit you choose to add)*
- Women : 2 tbsp chia seeds, ¾ cup almond milk ≅ 300-380 Calories *(based on the fruit you choose to add)*

Lunch : Chicken Caesar Salad

- Men : 150g chicken, 1 cup lettuce, 2 tbsp dressing ≅ 470 Calories
- Women : 100g chicken, 1 cup lettuce, 1 tbsp dressing ≅ 390 Calories

Dinner : Salmon Patty Burgers

- Men : 200g canned salmon, lettuce leaves as buns ≅ 500 Calories
- Women : 150g canned salmon, lettuce leaves as buns ≅ 390 Calories

Chapter 6:
PHYSICAL ACTIVITY GUIDELINES FOR ENDOMORPHS

***Note**: I do believe that this workout plan will help you tremendously achieve your fitness goals.*
However, if you're looking for something specifically tailored for your needs I suggest you write to this email: avfitness99coaching@gmail.com. Alessandro is an experienced personal trainer that wrote many books on fitness as well as having trained many people that struggle to lose weight. Contact him explaining you bought this book and you need some specific tips and guidance.

The Role of Exercise in Endomorph Weight Management

For endomorphs, who naturally have a slower metabolism and tend to carry more body fat, exercise isn't just beneficial—it's essential for effective weight management. The key to an effective exercise regimen for endomorphs lies in a mixture of two types of exercises:

1. ***Cardiovascular Fitness:*** Cardio exercises play a pivotal role in elevating heart rate and enhancing cardiorespiratory fitness. This includes two different subcategories: **HIIT** (High Intensity Interval Training) and **LISS** (Low-Intensity Steady State).
   This is particularly important for endomorphs as it aids in mitigating the risk of various health concerns, including cardiovascular diseases, obesity, hypertension, and type 2 diabetes.

2. ***Strength Training:*** Conversely, strength training is focused on building functional muscle mass, which in turn enhances metabolism and strength. This form of exercise is crucial for endomorphs because it helps you to lose

weight elevating the resting metabolic rate, meaning more calories are burned even when at rest as well as preserving muscle mass.

This combined method helps you lose weight, mainly in the form of body fat, while preserving muscle mass. Although it's not possible to lose only fat, this approach increases the amount of fat you lose compared to muscle.

The 4 Main Principles for Endomorph Fitness Routines

Based on experience, these are the best 4 guidelines to lose weight and improve your body composition, especially as an endomorph - This section is very important as I am going to outline the main strategies to get results. You can apply these to any training and obtain significant results as an endomorph.

- **Integrate HIIT**

In comparison to steady-state cardio, High-Intensity Interval Training (HIIT) effectively burns fat and improves cardiovascular health. Endomorphs can boost their metabolism and fat loss by including **two HIIT sessions per week**. It will simply be mixing up exercises where you do short bursts of activities at high intensity mixed with short breaks. You would repeat the sequence a few times.

The good thing about them is that it only takes 15-20 minutes to do them!

- **Focus on Compound Movements**

Squats, deadlifts, and overhead presses work out many muscles at once. If you're an endomorph, this can boost your metabolism by burning more calories and building muscle. It will also prevent the loss of muscle mass as it might occur when you're in caloric deficit.

Why do exercises that work many muscles at once? Because exercises that work only one muscle, like bicep curls and leg extensions, aren't worth your time. It's good for concentrating on one area, but it doesn't help burn calories as much.

Also, I will outline many exercises that works for most endomorphs as well as providing home variations in case you workout at home rather than in the gym)

- **Prioritize Functional Training**

Engaging in exercises that mimic everyday activities helps build strength where it counts, improving joint stability and reducing the risk of injury during high-impact exercises, which is particularly beneficial for endomorphs . That's why you will be doing lots of bodyweight movement that will not only make you sweat but improve your balance and coordination. Remember, you are training for long term benefits so it does not have to be all about calories. You should be a better "athlete" after these 12-weeks, not just with a few pounds less!

- **Embrace NEAT**

This is a crucial point that many training plans neglect. Yet, this is one of the most important things you can do to improve faster.

NEAT stands for Non-Exercise Activity Thermogenesis and It refers to the calories burned through daily activities outside of structured exercise or additional training sessions.
By taking walks and standing more, NEAT can be significantly increased, aiding in weight management.

What would that be in practice?

- Parking a bit further than usual so you walk a bit more.
- Taking stairs instead of the elevator.
- Spending less time sitting during the day.

Note: You will also perform on day a week of LISS (Low-Intensity Steady State) where you will do roughly 30-60 minutes of any type of cardio you like.
If on top of that you can have a general more active lifestyle, you will get results way quicker than you can imagine!

Calories Burnt in 60 Minutes of Activity

Exercise	Average Calories Burnt in an Hour
HIIT	600-900 Kcal
Jumping Rope	600-800 Kcal
Jogging	500-700 Kcal
Cycling	300-600 Kcal
Bodyweight Movement	300-350 Kcal
Strength Training	250-300 Kcal
Yoga	250 Kcal
Walking	150-200 Kcal

Exercise Timing for Endomorphs

For endomorphs, or anyone really, working out at the same time every day can make their exercise plan work better. This has two main advantages:

- First, it creates a routine that's easier to keep doing over time, which means you're more likely to stick with it.
- Second, it helps your body get into a rhythm with releasing certain hormones like cortisol and adrenaline at the same time every day, which is good for your workout.

A lot of people like working out in the morning because it gets your metabolism going early, helping you burn calories all day. But the most important thing is to pick a time that works for you, so you can keep it up regularly.

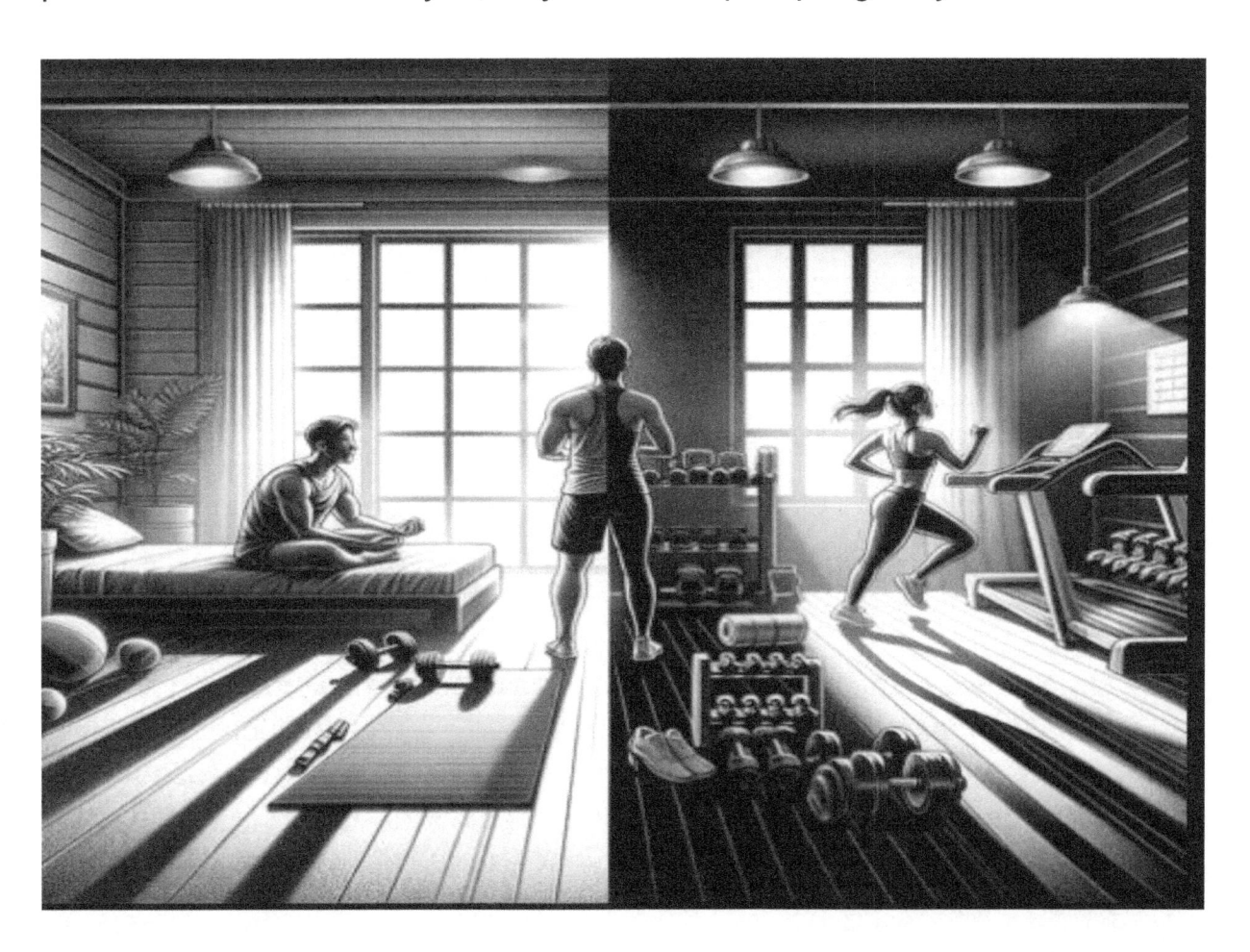

Chapter 7:
COMPREHENSIVE WORKOUT PROGRAMS

List of Exercises and How to Perform Them

LEGS

💪 Squats

How to:

- Stand with feet hip-width apart, toes slightly out. Arms on the side.
- Bend your knees and lower your hips as if sitting in a chair. Bring your hands together in front of your chest as you squat down.
- Once your thighs are parallel to the floor, pause for a moment and come back into the starting position pushing through your feets. Repeat for the mentioned reps.

Benefits : Strengthens quads, hamstrings, glutes, and core.

Beginner Modification : Limit the range of motion to make it easier.

Advanced Modification : Hold a dumbbell in front of your chest as you perform the movement.

Extra Notes: If you struggle with knee pain, make sure to do the lowering down part (eccentric phase) slowly. In fact, being able to execute the eccentric slowly is great for tendon health. Also, to make sure you are perfectly balanced when doing the movement, focus on three contact points of your feet to the floor: below the big toe, below the pinky and your heels. These three points apply pressure on the floor in equal measure at all times!

Glute Bridge

How to:
- Start by lying on your back on the floor with your knees bent and feet on the ground, hip-width apart. Place your arms at the side of your body
- From there. push through your heels to lift your hips off the ground towards the ceiling. Your body should form a straight line from your shoulders to your knees at the top of the movement.
- Pause at the top for one second, squeezing your glutes, then slowly lower your hips back to the starting position without touching the floor with your glutes..Repeat for the mentioned reps.

Benefits : It targets the glutes, but also works the hamstrings and core. It also helps in improving lower back strength and stability.

Beginner Modification _:_ Alternatively, you can perform the exercise with your feet elevated on a platform to reduce the range of motion.

Advanced Modification _:_ Add a plate or a sand bag at your hip level (hold it with your hands). As an alternative you can perform it single leg, lifting one leg off the ground and perform the exercise with only one foot pushing on the floor.

Extra Notes: some people tend to feel the front (or back) of their thighs when performing this exercise. If you are one of them, put extra pressure on your heels when squeezing your hips up. It will automatically engage more of your glutes.

Lunges

How to:
- Start with feet shoulder width apart and arms on the side.
- Step forward with one leg, lower your hips until both knees are bent at about a 90-degree angle. Keep the front knee above the ankle.
- Return to the starting position pushing with the front foot on the floor and repeat alternating the sides.

Benefits : Targets quads, hamstrings, glutes, and improves balance.

Beginner Modification : Limit the range of motion without going down too much.

Advanced Modification : Hold dumbbells on your hands for extra difficulty

Note: If you feel unstable when doing this movement I suggest you firstly do it barefoot when possible. The sensation of the foot on the floor will activate many dormant muscles of the foot that will help with balance. Then, I would recommend you to stare at a point a few feet in front of you on the floor. Having your sight fixed will help you increase your balance..

Step-Ups

How to:
- Face a bench or step.
- Step up with one foot, and push on the bench/step with your foot until you're standing on it.
- Then, step down, coming back to the starting position and repeatwith the other foot. Perform for the mentioned reps alternating the sides.

Benefits : Strengthens quads, hamstrings, and glutes; improves balance.

Beginner Modification : Use a lower step or bench to make it easier if you struggle with balance and/or strength.

Wall Sit

How to:

- Stand with your back against a wall, feet shoulder-width apart and.
- Slide your back down the wall, bending your knees to lower your body until your thighs are parallel to the floor, as if you were sitting in an invisible chair. Your knees should be directly above your ankles, and your back should stay against the wall.
- Hold this position for a set amount of time.

Benefits : Strengthens the quads, hamstrings, glutes, and calves as well as improving core stability.

Beginner Modification : If maintaining the parallel position is too challenging at first, don't slide down as far. Lower your body only as much as you can maintain without pain or discomfort.

Deadlifts

How to:

- Start with feet hip-width apart, hinge at the hips to bend over and grasp the bar (or dumbbells) keeping it close to your thighs/shins as you lower down.
- Feel the stretch on your hamstrings whilst keeping your back straight.
- Then, push through your heels to stand back up, engaging your glutes.
- Repeat for the mentioned reps.

Benefits : Works the posterior chain, including hamstrings, glutes, back, and core.

Beginner Modification : Use kettlebells or dumbbells with lighter weight.

Extra Note: It is important that as you lower down the barbell is very close to your shins. The closer it is to your body, the less pressure it will put on your lower back as well as engaging more your glutes.

Home Alternative : *Single-Leg Romanian Deadlifts (Bodyweight)*

How to:

- Stand on one leg, keeping a slight bend in the standing leg.
- Then, hinge at the hips to lower your trunk and reach your hands towards the floor, extending the other leg straight behind you for balance.
- Make sure to keep your back flat and head in a neutral position. Hold for a second and then come back into the starting position. Repeat on one side for 10 reps, then perform 10 reps with the other side. Perform 2 sets each side with no rest in between sets.

Benefits : it works the hamstrings, glutes, lower back, and core.. It simulates the deadlift's posterior chain engagement without needing external load (obviously, it is more balanced-focus than strength-focus as an exercise.

Beginner Modification : Perform the exercise near a wall or chair to lightly touch for balance if needed.

Kettlebell Swing

How to:

- Stand with feet wider than hip-width, holding a kettlebell with both hands (arms straight).
- Bend knees slightly, hinge at the hips to swing the kettlebell between your legs
- Then, using momentum, thrust hips forward to swing it up to chest height.
- Keep repeating the sequence at relatively high speed (once the technique is mastered).

Benefits : Improves posterior chain strength, cardiovascular endurance.

Beginner Modification : Start with a lighter weight and focus on form - avoid using your arms to generate power. The power comes from your legs and hips.

Home Alternative : **Squat Jump**

How to:

- Start standing with feet shoulder-width apart.
- Lower into a squat position. Keep your chest up and back straight. Bring your hands together in front of your chest
- Next, explosively jump up, pushing off the ground with your feet. Bring your arms next to your body as you do so (it will come naturally for most people anyway).
- Land softly back into the squat position to complete one rep. Aim to land gently, absorbing the impact. Repeat for the mentioned reps (the same mentioned for the Kettlebell Swing in the training plan.

Benefits *:* This exercise improves leg strength, explosiveness, and cardiovascular fitness. It targets many lower body muscles such as your quads, hamstrings, glutes, and calves.

Beginner Modification *:* If the jump is too challenging, perform a squat with just a small hop after that. As you get stronger, gradually work up to the full squat jump.

UPPER BODY

💪 Push-Ups

How to:

- Start in a plank position with arms straight, hands below your shoulder, slightly wider.
- Lower your body until your chest nearly touches the floor. Push through your arms to return to the starting position.

Benefits : Strengthens chest, shoulders, triceps, and core.Great exercise for upper body overall

Beginner Modification : Perform on knees or against a wall.

Advanced Modification : Lift your feet on a chair or step as you perform the push-up to make it more difficult in a simple yet effective way.

💪 Barbell Rows

How to:

- Start standing with feet shoulder width apart and gripping a barbell slightly wider than hid-width (both hands placement, facing you or in front of you, are okay)
- Bend forward at the waist, knees slightly bent,back and arms straight
- Pull the barbell towards your belly button, keeping the elbows close to the body.Squeeze your back for a second. Lower it back down. Repeat for the mentioned reps.

Benefits : Targets the back, shoulders, and biceps.

Beginner Modification : Use a lighter load or dumbbells instead. The movement would be the same but with dumbbells you will be able to move the weight with more ease (in fact, just the lightest bar in a commercial gym is around 15kg (30+ pounds) whilst you can start using dumbbells as heavy as 2.5kg (5 pounds).

Home Alternative: Floor Towel Lat Pulldown

How to:

- Lie on your back, legs straight, and hold a towel with both hands above your chest, arms straight.
- Keep tension in the towel as if you're trying to pull it apart.
- Lower your arms behind your head, keeping the tension in the towel.
- Then raise them back to the starting position. Repeat for 3 sets of 20 reps with 30 seconds rest in between,

Benefits : Targets the lats, shoulders, and improves shoulder mobility.

Bench Press

How to:

- Lie on a bench with feet planted on the ground. Grab the barbell wider than shoulder width. Keep your chest up as you perform the movement.
- Unrack the weight, and slowly control the bar until it almost touches your chest.
- Then, push the barbell up until your arms are straight. Lower it down again until it almost touches your chest, and then push it back up.
- Repeat for the mentioned reps.

Benefits : Strengthens chest, triceps, and shoulders.

Home Alternative: **Push-ups** (Explained before)

When done instead of the Bench Press, perform the same sets and reps mentioned for the bench press. Make it easier (on your knees) or more difficult (feet on a step) based on your fitness level.

Pull-Ups

How to:

- Hang from a pull-up bar with hands shoulder-width apart or slightly wider.
- Pull yourself up until your chin is over the bar, then lower back down.

Benefits : Works the back, shoulders, and biceps.

Beginner Modification : Use assisted pull-up machines or resistance bands, recommended for beginners

Home Alternative: *Floor Towel Lat Pulldown* (Explained before)

In case you perform this exercise instead of Pull-ups, perform 3 sets of 20 reps with 30 seconds rest in between

Overhead Press

How to:

- Stand with feet shoulder-width apart, holding a barbell at shoulder height. Press the weight up until arms are straight, then lower back to the starting position, repeating the sequence for the mentioned reps.

Benefits : Strengthens the shoulders, triceps, and core.

Beginner Modification : Use dumbbells for a lighter load.

Home Alternative: **Push-Ups** (Explained before)

When done instead of the Bench Press, perform the same sets and reps mentioned for the bench press. Make it easier (on your knees) or more difficult (feet on a step) based on your fitness level.

CORE

💪 Plank

How to:

- Hold a plank position with your forearms and toes on the floor, body in a straight line from head to heels, for the mentioned amount of seconds. Make sure not to arch your back.

Benefits : Strengthens the core, shoulders, and back. Improves posture and stability.

Beginner Modification : Perform the plank on your knees to reduce intensity.

Advanced Modification : Perform plank with your arms straight, only with the palms of your hands(and feet) on the floor. From there, lift one hand and touch the opposite shoulder, then put it back. Do the same with the other hand. Keep your body as still as a statue, only moving your hands. Repeat for the mentioned seconds

💪 Side Plank

How to:

- Lie on one side with your legs straight. Forearm and outside of the foot are in contact with the floor.
- Lift your hips to form a straight line from head to feet. Hold for the mentioned amount of seconds. Repeat on the other side.

Benefits : Targets the obliques, strengthening the side core muscles.

Beginner Modification : Bend your knees and perform the side plank from this position to lessen the difficulty.

Russian Twist

How to:

- Sit on the floor with knees bent, feet lifted slightly.
- Lean back slightly. Twist your torso to the right, then to the left, for the mentioned seconds.

Benefits : Strengthens and tones the abdominal muscles, especially the obliques. It also improves rotational mobility.

Beginner Modification : Keep feet on the floor to reduce the level of difficulty.

Leg Raises

How to:

- Lie on your back with legs straight and hands under your buttocks for support.
- Lift your legs to a 90-degree angle (vertical to the floor)
- Then, lower them without touching the floor. Repeat for the mentioned reps.

Benefits : Strengthens the lower abdominals and hip flexors. Improves core stability.

Beginner Modification : Bend your knees slightly as you raise and lower your legs to decrease the intensity.

CARDIO

💪 HIIT Sprints

How to:

Sprint at full effort for the mentioned seconds, then walk for the mentioned seconds.

Benefits : Boosts metabolism, improves cardiovascular health.
Beginner Modification: Reduce sprint time or intensity. Especially as a beginner do not sprint at 100% otherwise you might injure yourself.

Home Variation: *High-Knee Running in Place*

How to :

Run in place, lifting knees high, for the mentioned seconds. Rest for the given time - in case you do it instead of HIIT Sprints, perform it using the same time given on and off in the training plan.

Benefits : Increases heart rate, boosts metabolism, improves cardiovascular health.

Beginner Modification : Lower knee height and pace; gradually increase as fitness improves over the weeks.

💪 Jump Rope

How to:

With a rope, jump with both feet slightly off the ground. Keep jumps low to minimize impact. Keep doing it for the mentioned minutes taking as little breaks as possible.

Benefits: Improves cardiovascular fitness, leg strength, and coordination.

Rowing Machine

How to :

Sit on the rower, push with the legs first, then pull the handle towards your chest. Keep doing it for the mentioned seconds. In the HIIT sessions you'll be asked to perform a period of time at max speed and the following at slow pace, repeating the sequence a few times.

Benefits: Full-body workout, enhances cardiovascular endurance.

Beginner Modification: Use less resistance.

Home Alternative: **Jumping Jacks**

How to:

- Stand with your feet together and hands by your sides. Jump to a wider stance while raising your arms above your head, keeping them straight.
- Then quickly jump back to the starting position.
- Repeat the movement at a steady pace for 60 seconds, then rest 30" and repeat for 5 times. in total.

Benefits: Provides a full-body workout, similar to a rowing machine, by engaging multiple muscle groups.

Burpees

How to:

- From a standing position, drop into a squat, place hands on the ground, jump feet back into a plank, perform a push-up, jump feet back to squat, then jump up.

Benefits : Increases heart rate, works multiple muscle groups.

Beginner Modification : Walk back into plank instead of jumping and/or skip the push-up.

How to Warm-Up and Cool-Down Effectively

A proper warm-up and cool down are very important. Here is how you do them:

<u>A simple way to warm-up would be:</u>

Arm Circles (20 seconds each direction)

- Stand with your feet shoulder-width apart and extend your arms out to the sides at shoulder height.
- Make small circles with your arms.
- Reverse the direction after 20 seconds.

Leg Swings (10 swings per leg)

- Stand next to a wall or chair for support.
- Swing one leg forward and backward, keeping your posture upright.
- Repeat with the other leg.
-

Jumping Jacks (30 seconds low pace)

- Stand with your feet together and hands by your sides.
- Jump your feet out to the side while raising your arms above your head.
- Quickly jump back to the starting position. Repeat for 30 seconds warming up your body.
-

High Knees (30 seconds low pace)

- Stand with your feet hip-width apart.
- Jog in place, lifting your knees until your thigh is parallel to the floor.
- Pump your arms to increase the intensity, making it more realistic

<u>A simple way to warm-up would be:</u>

.Hamstring Stretch (30 seconds per leg)

- Stand and cross your right foot over your left.
- Slowly bend forward at the waist, keeping your legs straight, until you feel a gentle stretch along the back of your left leg.
- Hold for 30 seconds, then switch legs.

Quad Stretch (30 seconds per leg)

- Stand upright and pull your right foot towards your buttocks, holding it with your right hand.
- Keep your knees together and push your hips forward to enhance the stretch in your thigh.
- Hold for 30 seconds, then switch legs.

Arm & Shoulder Stretch (30 seconds per arm)

- Bring your right arm across your body at shoulder height.
- Use your left hand to gently press against your right arm, stretching the shoulder.
- Hold for 30 seconds, then switch arms.

Calf Stretch (30 seconds per leg)

- Stand facing a wall and place your right foot behind you, keeping it straight and pressing the heel into the floor.
- Bend your left knee and lean forward, keeping your back straight, until you feel a stretch in the calf of your back leg.
- Hold for 30 seconds, then switch legs.

Also, make sure to follow these four basic tips to stay in the game long enough and never get injured or be in pain that can take you out of training for weeks! (they will be repeated in Chapter 8 more extensively)

Listen to Your Body : Recognizing the difference between muscle fatigue and pain is crucial. If an exercise causes pain, stop immediately.

Increase Strength Gradually : Avoid jumping into high-intensity exercises without building foundational strength, especially around the joints, to prevent injuries .

Ensure Proper Technique : Always prioritize form over the amount of weight lifted or the speed of an exercise to avoid undue strain on the muscles and joints.

Rest and Recover : Adequate rest days are essential in allowing the body to recover and prevent overuse injuries, crucial for endomorphs who engage in frequent and intense workouts .

A 12-Week Fitness Schedule for Endomorphs

Notes Before you Start

Template : Each week you will have 5 sessions.
Two Strength training sessions (60 minutes long), two HIIT sessions (15-20 minutes long) and one light cardio session (30 to 60 minutes long).
You do not have to do them in any particular order. I lay out the plan in an "ideal way" but feel free to choose the order of the session you prefer the most. I recommend having a day off after strength training sessions as the next day you might be quite sore, especially at the beginning. However, fit the training based on your commitments and not vice versa (remember that consistency is key).

Strength Training Day : For each day I'm going to mention the name of the exercise (so you can look at the technique and notes I put on it), sets, reps and resting time between sets. Also I add a "Note" section to give you some extra tips for each exercise and /or explaining the progression. Remember to warm-up before the exercise (there's a quick warm-up routine in the last chapter). Do not go straight into the exercise plan otherwise you might get injured as your body is not ready to tolerate that stress without having warmed up first.

HIIT Session : As you can see, they only consist of two exercises. It is going to be short and intense so even if you are short of time, you can probably squeeze this session into your day. Make sure to warm up and cool down - especially before and after HIIT sessions, warming up and cooling down your body and heart rate is very very important.

Cardio Session : You will have plenty of choices for each time you do this workout. It will be anywhere between 30 and 60 minutes. If you have some extra time doing a few extra stretches once you finish would be very beneficial to relax your muscles. This session is quite important as it helps you burn calories making it easier to be in a caloric deficit

Deload Week : You will have two of them - one at Week 6 and one at Week 12, where you're going to do less intense routines. These weeks are useful to actively rest your body. You will still go to the gym but it's going to be a light session either because you do less sets per exercise, you do less reps per exercise or you use a lighter load - everything will be mentioned in the plan, no worries!

Extra Note : Also, there are some *Home Alternatives* in case you workout out at home rather than in the gym. For example, on a day you should do Bench Press, you can change it with Push-ups.

Bonus : In the plan from week 1 to week 2 I put progressions to make sure you constantly improve. The starting point is quite basic and for people who are not experienced with training. If you find that some progressions are too easy or your starting point in some exercises is higher than where the plan starts, please email avfitness99coaching@gmail.com so that you can get tailored advice!

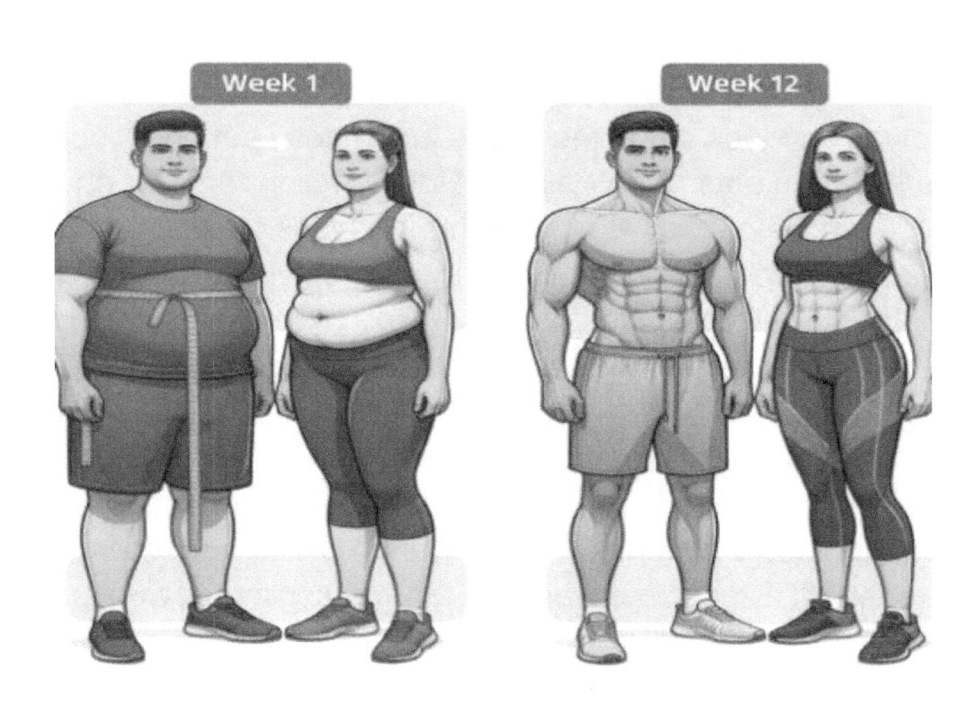

Week 1

Session 1 - Strength Training session

EXERCISE	SETS	REPS	REST	NOTE FOR BEGINNERS
Squats	4	8	60 seconds	Make sure to use a light load, especially in this first session.
Glute Bridge	3	12	30 seconds	Squeeze one second on top before coming back down.
Push Ups	4	8	60 seconds	If it's too difficult, go on your knees.
Barbell Rows	3	10	60 seconds	Start with a really light weight. Focusing on engaging your back each reps (elbows tucked in as you do the pulling).
Plank	2	30 seconds	30 seconds	Do not arch your back as you do that -Lower back should not be engaged.
Side Plank	1 (each side)	30 seconds	30 seconds	Start on your knees for the first time, unless you have done this exercise already.

Session 2 - HIIT session

Between HIIT Sprints and Jumping Rope take 2-3 minutes break.

EXERCISE	SETS AND REPS	NOTE
HIIT Sprint	20 second sprint, 40 second walk- repeat for 5 times	The sprint does not have to be 100% Start at 60/70% for this week
Jumping Rope	30 second on, 30 second off - Repeat for 5 times	try to be consistent for 30 seconds without stopping.

Session 3 - Strength Training session

EXERCISE	SETS	REPS	REST	NOTE
Lunges	4	14 (alternated)	30 seconds	Start doing it bodyweight
Step-Ups	2	20 (alternated)	60 seconds	Start doing it bodyweight
Bench Press	3	10	60 to 90 seconds	Do it with a light weight to start
Pull-Ups	4	5	60 to 90 seconds	Feel free to start with an assisted machine to start.
Russian Twist	3	30 seconds	30 seconds	Do the movement slowly to get the most out of it.
Leg Raises	2	10	30 seconds	Make sure to keep your core engaged at all times. You should not feel your lower back engaged

Session 4 - HIIT session

Between Rowing Machine and Burpees take 2-3 minutes break.

EXERCISE	SETS AND REPS	NOTE
Rowing Machine	20 seconds at 80% (almost max effort), 40 seconds at 20/30% (very low effort) - repeat for 5 times	Make sure to really change rhythm when you do the 20 seconds at high effort
Burpees	4 sets of 10 burpees, rest 60 seconds in between sets	Perform the beginner version (no push-ups and no jump) if you are not familiar with this exercise

Session 5

Choose between one of the following option:

- 40 minutes treadmill, medium pace walking, slightly inclined.
- 30 to 60 minutes walking outside medium to fast walking pace
- 45 minutes slow cycling
- 30 minutes Cross Trainer low intensity
- 25 to 35 minutes rowing machine low to medium intensity
- 20 minutes slow jogging either treadmill or outside

NEED EXTRA HELP? Send a video at avfitness99coaching@gmail.com and I'll assess your technique giving you tailored tips on how to make it better and safe!

Week 2

Session 1 - Strength Training session

EXERCISE	SETS	REPS	REST	NOTE
Squats	4	9	60 seconds	Add one more reps compared to last week, using the same load. (If you did it bodyweight, keep doing it bodyweight)
Glute Bridge	4	12	30 seconds	Let's do one more set today than last week!
Push Ups	4	8	60 seconds	No progression from last week. Make sure to master this exercise technique-wise
Barbell Rows	3	11-10-10	60 seconds	Let's add one more rep in the first set. Slow and constant progression is key!
Plank	2	45 seconds - 30 seconds	30 seconds	Try extending the first set of 15 seconds...I am sure you can do it!
Side Plank	1 (each side)	30 seconds	30 seconds	If you feel comfortable, do it the normal way on your feet. If not repeat it with your knees (and forearms, obviously) on the floor

Session 2 - HIIT session

Between HIIT Sprints and Jumping Rope take 2-3 minutes break.

EXERCISE	SETS AND REPS	NOTE
HIIT Sprint	25 second sprint, 35 second walk - Repeat for 5 times	In the 25 second slowly increase the speed
Jumping Rope	30 second on, 30 second off - Repeat for 5 times	try to be consistent for 30 seconds without stopping.

Session 3 - Strength Training session

EXERCISE	SETS	REPS	REST	NOTE
Deadlift	4	8	60 seconds	Choose a light load to master the technique first
Step-Ups	3	20 (alternated)	60 seconds	Add one more set from last week
Overhead Press	3	10	60 to 90 seconds	Do it with a light weight to start
Pull-Ups	4	5	60 to 90 seconds	Same as last week, use an assisted machine if you feel more comfortable.
Russian Twist	3	40 seconds	30 seconds	Increase the volume a bit adding extra seconds compared to last week
Leg Raises	2	12	30 seconds	Make sure to keep your core engaged at all times . You should not feel your lower back engaged

Session 4 - HIIT session

Between Rowing Machine and Burpees take 2-3 minutes break.

EXERCISE	SETS AND REPS	NOTE
Rowing Machine	25 seconds at 80% (almost max effort), 35 seconds at 20/30% (very low effort) - repeat for 5 times	Make sure, as mentioned last week to really push in the 25 seconds
Burpees	4 sets of 10 burpees, rest 60 seconds in between sets	Perform the beginner version (no push-ups and no jump) if you are not familiar with this exercise

Session 5

<u>Choose between one of the following option:</u>

- 40 minutes treadmill, medium pace walking, slightly inclined.
- 30 to 60 minutes walking outside medium to fast walking pace
- 45 minutes slow cycling
- 30 minutes Cross Trainer low intensity
- 25 to 35 minutes rowing machine low to medium intensity
- 20 minutes slow jogging either treadmill or outside

Week 3

Session 1 - Strength Training session

EXERCISE	SETS	REPS	REST	NOTE
Squats	4	10	60 seconds	Make sure to keep the technique spot on as we progress the number of reps
Glute Bridge	4	12	30 seconds	No tips needed
Push Ups	4	9-9-8-8	60 seconds	Let's add one more rep in the first two sets!
Barbell Rows	4	11	60 seconds	Big improvement here. Let's do 4 sets. By week 3 you should be able to engage your back as you do so. If not email avfitness99coaching@gmail.com and he will be able to guide you more"
Plank	2	45 seconds	30 seconds	Both sets are 45 seconds!
Side Plank	2 (each side)	30 seconds	30 seconds	Let's increase the volume adding one more sets for each side

Session 2 - HIIT session

Between HIIT Sprints and Jumping Rope take 2-3 minutes break.

EXERCISE	SETS AND REPS	NOTE
HIIT Sprint	25 second sprint, 35 second walk - Repeat for 5 times	In the 25 second slowly increase the speed up to 80/90%
Jumping Rope	40 second on, 20 second off - Repeat for 5 times	Increased working time now

Session 3 - Strength Training session

EXERCISE	SETS	REPS	REST	NOTE
Lunges	4	18 (alternated)	30 seconds	Perform it bodyweight
Step-Ups	3	20 (alternated)	60 seconds	Add one more set from last week
Bench Press	3	11	60 to 90 seconds	Increase the reps from Week 1 whilst keeping the same load
Pull-Ups	4	5	60 to 90 seconds	Same as last week, use an assisted machine if you feel more comfortable.
Russian Twist	3	40 seconds	30 seconds	Increase the volume a bit adding extra seconds compared to last week
Leg Raises	2	15	30 seconds	15 reps would be a very good standard…well done if you can complete it with ease!

Session 4 - HIIT session

Between Rowing Machine and Burpees take 2-3 minutes break

EXERCISE	SETS AND REPS	NOTE
Rowing Machine	25 seconds at 80% (almost max effort), 35 seconds at 20/30% (very low effort) - repeat for 5 times	Make sure to really push in the 25 seconds
Burpees	4 sets of 10 burpees, rest 50 seconds in between sets	Let's decrease resting time now!

Session 5

Choose between one of the following option:

- 40 minutes treadmill, medium pace walking, slightly inclined.
- 30 to 60 minutes walking outside medium to fast walking pace
- 45 minutes slow cycling
- 30 minutes Cross Trainer low intensity
- 25 to 35 minutes rowing machine low to medium intensity
- 20 minutes slow jogging either treadmill or outside

Week 4

Session 1 - Strength Training session

EXERCISE	SETS	REPS	REST	NOTE
Squats	4	8	60 seconds	Increase the weight now! Add 5 to 10 pounds and see how it goes! Start with a 15-20 pound dumbbell holding it in front of your chest if you did only bodyweight before.
Glute Bridge	4	12	30 seconds	Increase the weight of 5 to 10 pounds! If you did it bodyweight before, start with a 15-20 pounds dumbbell or sandbag on your hips.
Push Ups	4	9-9-8-8	60 seconds	Same as last week, you should be able to complete it now with ease!
Barbell Rows	4	12	60 seconds	No tips needed, simply adding one rep for each set, keeping the same load
Plank	2	60 seconds - 45 seconds	30 seconds	Well done! Let's try 60 seconds for the first set
Side Plank	2 (each side)	45 seconds - 30 seconds	30 seconds	Slightly increase in volume here for the first set.

Session 2 - HIIT session

Between HIIT Sprints and Jumping Rope take 2-3 minutes break.

EXERCISE	SETS AND REPS	NOTE
HIIT Sprint	25 second sprint, 35 second walk - Repeat for 6 times	Add one more set
Jumping Rope	40 second on, 20 second off- Repeat for 6 times	

Session 3 - Strength Training session

EXERCISE	SETS	REPS	REST	NOTE
Lunges	4	18 (alternated)	30 seconds	Last week of doing it bodyweight
Step-Ups	3	12 (alternated)	60 seconds	Use two dumbbells of 10 pounds each when doing the movement
Overhead Press	3	11	60 to 90 seconds	Increase the reps from Week 2 whilst keeping the same load
Pull-Ups	4	5	60 to 90 seconds	Same as last week, use an assisted machine if you feel more comfortable.
Russian Twist	2	50 seconds	30 seconds	No tips needed
Leg Raises	2	15	30 seconds	15 reps would eb a very good standard…well done if you can complete it with ease!

Session 4 - HIIT session

Between Rowing Machine and Burpees take 2-3 minutes break.

EXERCISE	SETS AND REPS	NOTE
Rowing Machine	25 seconds at 80% (almost max effort), 35 seconds at 20/30% (very low effort) - repeat for 6 times	Let's increase to 6 sets
Burpees	4 sets of 10 burpees, rest 50 seconds in between sets	

Session 5

<u>Choose between one of the following option:</u>

- 40 minutes treadmill, medium pace walking, slightly inclined.
- 30 to 60 minutes walking outside medium to fast walking pace
- 45 minutes slow cycling
- 30 minutes Cross Trainer low intensity
- 25 to 35 minutes rowing machine low to medium intensity
- 20 minutes slow jogging either treadmill or outside

Week 5

Session 1 - Strength Training session

EXERCISE	SETS	REPS	REST	NOTE
Squats	4	9	60 seconds	Increase the reps keeping the same weight you used before.
Glute Bridge	4	12	30 seconds	Same as last week, master the technique.
Push Ups	4	9	60 seconds	Let's do 9 reps for each set now! make sure to revisit the technique in the tutorial to perform it right.
Barbell Rows	4	9	60 seconds	Increase the load of 10-15 pounds
Plank	2	60 seconds - 45 seconds	30 seconds	No tips needed
Side Plank	2 (each side)	45 seconds - 30 seconds	30 seconds	No tips needed

Session 2 - HIIT session

Between HIIT Sprints and Jumping Rope take 2-3 minutes break.

EXERCISE	SETS AND REPS
HIIT Sprint	30 second sprint, 30 second walk - Repeat for 6 times
Kettlebell Swing	12 reps with light load (15-20 pounds), rest 30". Repeat 5 times

Session 3 - Strength Training session

EXERCISE	SETS	REPS	REST	NOTE
Deadlift	4	10	60 seconds	Same Load of Week 3, but more reps in
Step-Ups	3	12 (alternated)	60 seconds	Same as last week
Bench Press	3	12	60 to 90 seconds	Increase the reps from Week 1 whilst keeping the same load
Pull-Ups	4	5	60 to 90 seconds	If you feel comfortable, try using an elastic band to make it slightly more challenging than doing it with an assisted machine.
Russian Twist	2	50 seconds	30 seconds	No tips needed
Leg Raises	2	15	30 seconds	

Session 4 - HIIT session

Between Rowing Machine and Burpees take 2-3 minutes break.

EXERCISE	SETS AND REPS
Rowing Machine	25 seconds at 80% (almost max effort), 35 seconds at 20/30% (very low effort) - repeat for 6 times
Burpees	4 sets of 10 burpees, rest 40 seconds in between sets

Session 5

<u>Choose between one of the following option:</u>

- 40 minutes treadmill, medium pace walking, slightly inclined.
- 30 to 60 minutes walking outside medium to fast walking pace
- 45 minutes slow cycling
- 30 minutes Cross Trainer low intensity
- 25 to 35 minutes rowing machine low to medium intensity
- 20 minutes slow jogging either treadmill or outside

Week 6 - Deload Week

Session 1 - Strength Training session

EXERCISE	SETS	REPS	REST	NOTE - Let's decrease number of sets to make sure you do a light session that make you feel better without tiring yourself out
Squats	2	9	60 seconds	Sme load of last week
Glute Bridge	2	12	30 seconds	Same load of last week
Push Ups	2	9	60 seconds	No tips needed
Barbell Rows	2	9	60 seconds	Same load of last week
Plank	1	60 seconds		No tips needed
Side Plank	1 (each side)	45 seconds		No tips needed

Session 2 - HIIT session

Between HIIT Sprints and Jumping Rope take 2-3 minutes break.

EXERCISE	SETS AND REPS	NOTE
HIIT Sprint	30 second sprint, 30 second walk - Repeat for 2 times	Easy week, not much volume
Jumping Rope	40 second on, 20 second off - Repeat for 3 times	

Session 3 - Strength Training session (decrease load or reps here no sets)

Lunges	2	12 (alternated)	30 seconds	Bodyweight
Step-Ups	3	12 (alternated)	60 seconds	Bodyweight
Overhead press	3	8	60 to 90 seconds	Same load of week 3, decrease reps
Pull-Ups	2	5	60 to 90 seconds	If you feel comfortable, try using an elastic band to make it slightly more challenging than doing it with an assisted machine.
Russian Twist	2	50 seconds	30 seconds	
Leg Raises	2	10	30 seconds	

Session 4 - HIIT session

Between Rowing Machine and Burpees take 2-3 minutes break.

EXERCISE	SETS AND REPS
Rowing Machine	25 seconds at 80% (almost max effort), 35 seconds at 20/30% (very low effort) - Repeat for 3 times
Burpees	2 sets of 10 burpees, rest 60 seconds in between sets

Session 5

<u>Choose between one of the following option:</u>

- 40 minutes treadmill, medium pace walking, slightly inclined.
- 30 to 60 minutes walking outside medium to fast walking pace
- 45 minutes slow cycling
- 30 minutes Cross Trainer low intensity
- 25 to 35 minutes rowing machine low to medium intensity
- 20 minutes slow jogging either treadmill or outside

Week 7

Session 1 - Strength Training session

EXERCISE	SETS	REPS	REST	NOTE
Squats	4	9	60 seconds	No tips needed
Glute Bridge	4	8	30 seconds	Increase the load of 15-20 pounds
Push Ups	4	10-9-9-9	60 seconds	By now you should do most reps without knee assistance, if so…well done!
Barbell Rows	4	10	60 seconds	Keep the same load whilst adding one more reps. Make sure each rep is executed with perfect technique
Plank	2	60 seconds - 45 seconds	30 seconds	No tips needed
Side Plank	2 (each side)	45 seconds	30 seconds	Increase to 45 seconds for every set you do

Session 2 - HIIT session

Between HIIT Sprints and Jumping Rope take 2-3 minutes break.

EXERCISE	SETS AND REPS
HIIT Sprint	30 second sprint, 30 second walk - Repeat for 7 times
Jumping Rope	50 second on, 10 second off - Repeat for 5 times

Session 3 - Strength Training session

EXERCISE	SETS	REPS	REST	NOTE
Lunges	2	14 (alternated)	30 seconds	Use two dumbbells of 10 pounds each when doing the movement
Step-Ups	3	12 (alternated)	60 seconds	Same as last week
Bench Press	3	9	60 to 90 seconds	Increase the load of 15-20 pounds
Pull-Ups	4	6	60 to 90 seconds	If you feel comfortable, try using an elastic band to make it slightly more challenging than doing it with an assisted machine.
Russian Twist	2	60 seconds	30 seconds	
Leg Raises	2	18	30 seconds	

Session 4 - HIIT session

Between Rowing Machine and Burpees take 2-3 minutes break.

EXERCISE	SETS AND REPS
Rowing Machine	30 seconds at 80% (almost max effort), 30 seconds at 20/30% (very low effort) - Repeat for 6 times
Burpees	3 sets of 12 burpees, rest 40 seconds in between sets

Session 5

<u>Choose between one of the following option:</u>

- 40 minutes treadmill, medium pace walking, slightly inclined.
- 30 to 60 minutes walking outside medium to fast walking pace
- 45 minutes slow cycling
- 30 minutes Cross Trainer low intensity
- 25 to 35 minutes rowing machine low to medium intensity
- 20 minutes slow jogging either treadmill or outside

Week 8

Session 1 - Strength Training session

EXERCISE	SETS	REPS	REST	NOTE
Squats	4	10-10-9-9	60 seconds	Slightly increase of reps with the same load
Glute Bridge	4	8	30 seconds	Same as last week, manage the last week's weight with perfect technique squeezing the glutes on top after each rep.
Push Ups	4	10-9-9-9	60 seconds	No tips needed
Barbell Rows	4	10	60 seconds	No tips needed
Plank	2	60 seconds	30 seconds	2 sets of 60 seconds was the end goal of this plan, well done!
Side Plank	1 (each side)	60 seconds	30 seconds	let's do only one set and push it to 60 seconds…if you cannot, no worries. Try your best though!

Session 2 - HIIT session

Remember to take 2-3 minutes between HIIT Sprints and Jumping Rope

EXERCISE	SETS AND REPS
HIIT Sprint	30 second sprint, 30 second walk - repeat for 7 times
Jumping Rope	5 minutes non stop - (ideally)

Session 3 - Strength Training session

EXERCISE	SETS	REPS	REST	NOTE
Lunges	2	14 (alternated)	30 seconds	Use 10 pounds dumbbells on each side
Deadlift	4	8	60 seconds	increase weight of 20 pounds
Overhead Press	3	9	60 to 90 seconds	Increase the load of 10-15 pounds from what you did before
Pull-Ups	4	6	60 to 90 seconds	If you feel comfortable, try using an elastic band to make it slightly more challenging than doing it with an assisted machine.
Russian Twist	2	60 seconds	30 seconds	
Leg Raises	2	18	30 seconds	

Session 4 - HIIT session

Between Rowing Machine and Burpees take 2-3 minutes break.

EXERCISE	SETS AND REPS
Rowing Machine	30 seconds at 80% (almost max effort), 30 seconds at 20/30% (very low effort) - Repeat for 6 times
Kettlebell Swing	15 reps with light load (15-20 pounds), rest 30". Repeat 5 times

Session 5

<u>Choose between one of the following option:</u>

- 40 minutes treadmill, medium pace walking, slightly inclined.
- 30 to 60 minutes walking outside medium to fast walking pace
- 45 minutes slow cycling
- 30 minutes Cross Trainer low intensity
- 25 to 35 minutes rowing machine low to medium intensity
- 20 minutes slow jogging either treadmill or outside

Week 9

Session 1 - Strength Training session

EXERCISE	SETS	REPS	REST	NOTE
Squats	4	10	60 seconds	4 sets of 10, well done!
Glute Bridge	4	9	30 seconds	Add one rep in every set. Keep the same load
Push Ups	4	10-9-9-9	60 seconds	No tips needed
Barbell Rows	4	11	60 seconds	Let's build the volume, next week we'll add more load!
Plank	2	60 seconds	30 seconds	If too easy look at "advanced modification" in the Plank explanation
Side Plank	1 (each side)	60 seconds	30 seconds	

Session 2 - HIIT session

Remember to take 2-3 minutes between HIIT Sprints and Jumping Rope

EXERCISE	SETS AND REPS
HIIT Sprint	30 second sprint, 30 second walk - Repeat for 8 times
Jumping Rope	5 minutes non stop - (ideally)

Session 3 - Strength Training session

EXERCISE	SETS	REPS	REST	NOTE
Lunges	2	16 (alternated)	30 seconds	Use 10 pounds dumbbells on each side
Step-Ups	3	14 (alternated)	60 seconds	Use 10 pounds dumbbells on each side
Bench Press	4	9	60 to 90 seconds	Same weight of Week 7 Increase number of sets from three to four
Pull-Ups	4	6	60 to 90 seconds	If you feel comfortable, try using an elastic band to make it slightly more challenging than doing it with an assisted machine.
Russian Twist	2	60 seconds	30 seconds	
Leg Raises	2	18	30 seconds	

Session 4 - HIIT session

Between Rowing Machine and Burpees take 2-3 minutes break.

EXERCISE	SETS AND REPS
Rowing Machine	30 seconds at 90% (close to max effort), 30 seconds at 20/30% (very low effort) - repeat for 7 times
Burpees	3 sets of 12 burpees, rest 30 seconds in between sets

Session 5

<u>Choose between one of the following option:</u>

- 40 minutes treadmill, medium pace walking, slightly inclined.
- 30 to 60 minutes walking outside medium to fast walking pace
- 45 minutes slow cycling
- 30 minutes Cross Trainer low intensity
- 25 to 35 minutes rowing machine low to medium intensity
- 20 minutes slow jogging either treadmill or outside

Week 10

Session 1 - Strength Training session

EXERCISE	SETS	REPS	REST	NOTE
Squats	3	11	60 seconds	Same load of last week
Glute Bridge	4	9	30 seconds	
Push Ups	4	10-9-9-9	60 seconds	No tips needed
Barbell Rows	4	8	60 seconds	Add roughly 10 pounds on the barbell
Plank	3	60 seconds	30 seconds	
Side Plank	1 (each side)	60 seconds	30 seconds	

Session 2 - HIIT session

Remember to take 2-3 minutes between HIIT Sprints and Jumping Rope

EXERCISE	SETS AND REPS
HIIT Sprint	30 second sprint, 30 second walk - Repeat for 9 times
Jumping Rope	5 minutes non stop - (ideally)

Session 3 - Strength Training session

EXERCISE	SETS	REPS	REST	NOTE
Lunges	3	16 (alternated)	30 seconds	Increase number of sets, same load.
Step-Ups	3	14 (alternated)	60 seconds	
Overhead Press	4	9	60 to 90 seconds	Same weight of Week 8 Increase number of sets from three to four
Pull-Ups	3	7	60 to 90 seconds	If you feel comfortable, try using an elastic band to make it slightly more challenging than doing it with an assisted machine.
Russian Twist	3	60 seconds	30 seconds	
Leg Raises	2	20	30 seconds	

Session 4 - HIIT session

Between Rowing Machine and Burpees take 2-3 minutes break.

EXERCISE	SETS AND REPS
Rowing Machine	30 seconds at 90% (close to max effort), 30 seconds at 20/30% (very low effort) - Repeat for 8 times
Burpees	3 sets of 12 burpees, rest 15 seconds in between sets

Session 5

<u>Choose between one of the following option:</u>

- 40 minutes treadmill, medium pace walking, slightly inclined.
- 30 to 60 minutes walking outside medium to fast walking pace
- 45 minutes slow cycling
- 30 minutes Cross Trainer low intensity
- 25 to 35 minutes rowing machine low to medium intensity
- 20 minutes slow jogging either treadmill or outside

Week 11

Session 1 - Strength Training session

EXERCISE	SETS	REPS	REST	NOTE
Squats	4	11	60 seconds	Add one more set
Glute Bridge	4	9	30 seconds	
Push Ups	4	10-9-9-9	60 seconds	No tips needed
Barbell Rows	4	8	60 seconds	Same load of last week
Plank	3	60 seconds	30 seconds	
Side Plank	2 (each side)	60 seconds	30 seconds	

Session 2 - HIIT session

Remember to take 2-3 minutes between HIIT Sprints and Jumping Rope

EXERCISE	SETS AND REPS
HIIT Sprint	30 second sprint, 30 second walk - Repeat for 10 times
Kettlebell Swing	15 reps with light load (15-20 pounds), rest 30". Repeat 6 times

Session 3 - Strength Training session

EXERCISE	SETS	REPS	REST	NOTE
Lunges	3	16 (alternated)	30 seconds	Increase number of sets, same load.
Deadlift	4	10	60 seconds	Increased reps, managing the same load of last time.
Bench Press	4	10	60 to 90 seconds	Same weight of week 9 but one more rep for each set, make sure the technique is spot on
Pull-Ups	3	5-5-x	60 to 90 seconds	The first two sets do only 5 reps. In the last set try performing one unassisted pull ups, let's see where you're at!
Russian Twist	2	60 seconds	30 seconds	Use a 2-4kg (less than 10 pounds) medicine ball and hold it at chest level. Rotate whilst holding the ball.
Leg Raises	2	20	30 seconds	

Session 4 - HIIT session

Between Rowing Machine and Burpees take 2-3 minutes break.

EXERCISE	SETS AND REPS
Rowing Machine	30 seconds at 90% (close to max effort), 30 seconds at 20/30% (very low effort) - Repeat for 9 times
Burpees	25 burpees non stop, one set only

Session 5

<u>Choose between one of the following option:</u>

- 40 minutes treadmill, medium pace walking, slightly inclined.
- 30 to 60 minutes walking outside medium to fast walking pace
- 45 minutes slow cycling
- 30 minutes Cross Trainer low intensity
- 25 to 35 minutes rowing machine low to medium intensity
- 20 minutes slow jogging either treadmill or outside

Week 12- Deload Week

Session 1 - Strength Training session

EXERCISE	SETS	REPS	REST	NOTE
Squats	4	12	30 seconds	Do it bodyweight
Glute Bridge	4	15	30 seconds	Do it bodyweight
Push Ups	4	5	30 seconds	
Plank	1	60 seconds		
Side Plank	1 (each side)	60 seconds	30 seconds	

Session 2

Day off, no HIIT session today. If you want to do some yoga or stretching.

Session 3 - Strength Training session

EXERCISE	SETS	REPS	REST	NOTE
Lunges	3	20 (alternated)	30 seconds	Bodyweight
Step-Ups	3	20 (alternated)	60 seconds	Bodyweight
Overhead Press	2	10	60 to 90 seconds	Same load you used on week 10, just one more rep each set and 2 sets only.
Pull-Ups	2	5-5	60 to 90 seconds	Use an elastic band (if not comfortable use unassisted pull-ups)
Russian Twist	2	30 seconds	15 to 30 seconds	Bodyweight
Leg Raises	2	10	30 seconds	

Session 4 - Between Rowing Machine and Burpees take 2-3 minutes break.

EXERCISE	SETS AND REPS
Rowing Machine	30 seconds at 90% (close to max effort), 30 seconds at 20/30% (very low effort) - Repeat for 4 times
Burpees	2 sets of 12 burpees, rest 60 seconds

Session 5

Choose between one of the following option:

- 40 minutes treadmill, medium pace walking, slightly inclined.
- 30 to 60 minutes walking outside medium to fast walking pace
- 45 minutes slow cycling
- 30 minutes Cross Trainer low intensity
- 25 to 35 minutes rowing machine low to medium intensity
- 20 minutes slow jogging either treadmill or outside

Chapter 8:
REST, RECOVERY, AND REJUVENATION

To feel good and active, it is essential to implement effective rest and recovery strategies. Here's a step-by-step guide to incorporating these practices into your daily life.

Note: These tips are quite general. There's no specific best form of recovery for endomorphs, so while I recommend checking them out, you might already be familiar with this advice!

Integrating Rest into Your Wellness Routine

Plan Your Rest Days: Have at least one or two days each week exclusively for rest, marking them on your calendar as non-negotiable rest days. By doing so your body gets the necessary time to heal and be ready for the next workouts.

Listen to Your Body: Pay close attention to your body's feedback. It does not mean that if you feel slightly sore today, tomorrow you do not workout. It means that if you have joint pain you do less or simply work around the pain (imagine you have elbow pain: you still workout but simply avoid exercises that put stress on it such as push-ups or bench press).

Note: as mentioned previously, email avfitness99coaching@gmail.com explaining your training situation and he can help you figure out the best way to approach your situation.

Enhancing Recovery with Practical Strategies

- **Active Recovery Activities**

Incorporate gentle activities like walking ,ideally outside but readmill works well too), participating in a yoga class, or enjoying a casual bike ride. These low-intensity activities boost blood flow, speeding up the recovery.

(Yes, I hate to break it to you but laying on the couch is not a great form of recovery!)

Action you can take: At least twice per week go for a short walk of 10-20 minutes in a park, while listening to music or chatting with friends.

- **Post-Workout Nutrition**

Prioritize a balanced intake of protein and carbohydrates shortly after exercising. Also, make sure to get antioxidants in. Great sources are berries (especially blueberries), broccoli and cauliflower.

Action you can take: As a snack you might want to consider, at least on most days, adding strawberries or blueberries.

- **Hydration Focus**

Drink water all day long to help your body heal itself.. The days of training try drinking slightly more around the workout. These little yet effective guidelines will help you more than you think.

Action you can take: Try to drink at least a sip of water every hour from the time you wake up to 2-3 hours before you go to sleep.

- **Daily Mobility Practices**

10 to 15 minutes for foam rolling and stretching exercises, concentrating on sore or tight areas will help you tremendously.Any Youtube routine works well.

Action you can take: *Simply write "Stretching Routine", "Yoga Routine to Relax your body" or "Myofascial Release" and pick any 10-15 minute routine you like at least once a week.*

Stress Management and Sleep Improvement Techniques

Establish a Pre-Sleep Ritual: Create a relaxing routine before bedtime to transition your body and mind into sleep mode. Reading a fiction book, journaling about the day, meditating, or taking a warm bath can effectively calm your senses. Avoid electronic devices to minimize blue light exposure that can have a negative impact on sleep.

Optimize Your Sleeping Environment: Make your bedroom cool, dark, and quiet. Use blackout curtains, earplugs, or white noise machines as needed, and invest in a high-quality mattress and pillows for maximal comfort. Quality sleep is even more important than quantity!

Mindfulness and Meditation: Reserve a few moments each day for mindfulness practices or meditation to alleviate stress and promote better sleep. Utilize guided sessions from applications like Headspace or Calm to ease into a peaceful state of mind. Simply 5 minutes per day where you observe your breath or pay attention to a particular point of your body will make you more calm and centered as well as making you fall asleep faster.

Chapter 9:
EASY-TO-READ GUIDE ON SUPPLEMENTAL SUPPORT FOR ENDOMORPHS

Adding certain supplements to what you eat every day can help a lot. They can make your metabolism faster, help you lose fat, and help you build muscle. Just remember, these supplements are just "supplements" to go with eating healthy and exercising often, not things to use instead of them.

Note: Some advice here has been already given in chapter 3, especially concerning Zinc, Magnesium and Vitamin D.

Protein Powder

Eating enough protein is important for repairing muscles and feeling full until your next meal. Putting a scoop of protein powder in your shakes (shakes can be a good snack on workout days) can make your muscles stronger and help you not want to snack so much. If dairy products don't feel good to you, you can try protein from plants like soy, almond or rice milk instead!

Why is this important for endomorphs? Muscle maintenance and satiety are key for endomorphs to efficiently manage weight and body composition, avoiding overeating carbs and fats.

Fish Oil (Omega-3s)

Omega-3s can help make your body better at using sugars from your food, so you store less fat. They're also great for reducing inflammation, helping your body recover faster from workouts.

Why is this important for endomorphs? Endomorphs benefit from omega-3s as these fatty acids help counteract their predisposition towards insulin resistance and inflammation-related recovery delays. This helps for a healthier metabolism and more effective fat loss over time.

Green Tea Extract

This supplement can give your metabolism a little boost, helping your body burn more calories even when you're not working out. Also, it's a nice, gentle way to get a bit of extra energy without the jitters. I will suggest you to avoid it after 3pm because it contains a bit of caffeine that might have a harmful impact on your sleep.

Why is this important for endomorphs? Given the naturally lower basal metabolic rate of endomorphs, any safe and sustainable boost to metabolism, like that from green tea extract, can significantly impact your ability to lose weight as well as improving your energy levels.

Magnesium

This essential mineral supports muscle and nerve function and is vital for energy production. Magnesium can help improve sleep quality, which is crucial for muscle recovery and hormonal balance, making it a beneficial supplement for endomorphs.

Why is this important for endomorphs? Since endomorphs can easily accumulate fat due to hormonal imbalances and stress, magnesium's ability to improve sleep and subsequently balance hormones makes it an important supplement for this body type's overall health and weight management.

Vitamin D

Often overlooked, Vitamin D, as mentioned before, is crucial for bone health, immune function, and may even aid in weight loss by influencing the way your body stores fat. Since obtaining enough Vitamin D from food alone can be challenging, supplementation can be particularly helpful, especially in less sunny locales.

Why is this important for endomorphs? Ensuring optimal levels of Vitamin D is crucial for endomorphs as it supports the hormonal balance and metabolic functions needed to overcome their natural inclination towards storing fat, particularly in challenging to lose areas.

Zinc

As mentioned in chapter 3, Zinc is very important for regulating metabolism, balancing hormones (including testosterone, which is crucial for muscle building), and optimizing your immune system. In fact, Improved metabolic rate aids in burning more calories, hormone balance is critical for weight and health management, and a strong immune system supports consistent training schedules without getting sick, and therefore having to pause your exercise routine.

Why is this specifically important for endomorphs? *Zinc supports the critical areas of metabolism, hormonal health, and immune function, directly impacting endomorphs' ability to manage their weight, build muscle, and maintain overall health, making it a great supplement especially if you do not take enough zinc from food*

FAQs

1. "Do I really have an endomorph body type, and why does it matter?"

If you find it easy to gain weight but hard to lose it, you might be an endomorph. Understanding this can help you choose the right food and exercises for your body, instead of just doing what others do.

It's about helping your body be its best, not fighting with it. Understanding your body type means recognizing that you may benefit more from steady state training (SST), like walking, jogging, or swimming, in addition to the exercises and diet advice given in this book. This book treats diet and exercises exactly for endomorphs, so no worries, I got you covered!

2. "What's the secret to dieting for someone like me?"

Imagine this: Instead of stopping eating all carbs and feeling unhappy, you make your meals with a good mix of lean proteins, vegetables full of fiber, and a little bit of whole grains (In the 28-Day Plan I'll give you specific guidelines). It's not about following tough rules but making a way of eating that you can keep doing consistently, which helps you stay full and full of energy.

3. "I hate running. What exercises are actually good for endomorphs?"

Think about making your metabolism faster without needing to run on a treadmill for a long time. If you're an endomorph, incorporating a variety of workouts, including HIIT for short, intense exercises, and also steady state training (SST) for longer sessions (you will be doing once a week this type of session) of moderate to low intensity, can be highly beneficial. Also, lifting weights or doing exercises to make your muscles stronger helps your body keep burning calories even when you're not working out.

Be sure to follow the plan as it comprehends compound exercises like squats, deadlifts, presses, and rows in your routine. I will also leave you room for choosing the exercises you prefer; from home variations (push-ups instead of bench press) to different cardio exercises you can do.

Exercising should make you feel good, not like you're being punished. In the 12-week training routine, I outline the best strategies for endomorphs, emphasizing the importance of both cardiovascular and strength training exercises- It worked for many people before you, so I am confident it will help you too!

4. "Exercise every day? How realistic is that?"

Imagine it like this: Endomorphs aiming for fat loss and improved body composition should consider engaging in exercise 5 to 6 days per week, for 30 to 60 minutes, depending on fitness levels and workout intensity. Some days, you might lift weights or do a HIIT workout for a short time. On other days, you might go for a long walk, stretch, or do yoga. It's all about moving your body, not just doing strenuous workouts. In the 12-week plan I did my best to tailored a workout that does all of this!

5. "Can I still enjoy carbs or should I say goodbye forever?"

Imagine enjoying a sweet potato or quinoa without guilt. As an endomorph, focusing on low-glycemic carbohydrates that don't spike your blood sugar is crucial. It's about choosing carbs that offer more than just calories—think about fiber, vitamins, and minerals.. You do not have to remove carbs; you simply have to redirect your meals to healthier options.

6. "Why is protein such a big deal?"

Imagine protein as the main ingredient for making your muscles strong. After you exercise, eating something with a lot of protein helps fix and build up your muscles. Also, it's like a special trick for not getting hungry quickly—it helps you stay full, which makes following your eating plan easier without eating ezra snacks outside your meals.

7. "Are supplements really necessary?"

While whole foods should always be the star of your diet, think of supplements as the supporting cast. A protein powder can be a convenient post-workout snack, and omega-3s from fish oil might help with inflammation. They're not must-haves but can complement a well-rounded diet.

8. "How can I rev up my slow metabolism?"

Beyond exercise, small lifestyle tweaks can add up. Consider the thermogenic effect of food—spicy dishes can temporarily boost metabolism. Even staying hydrated plays a role; think of water as fuel for your metabolic fire. These are not life-changing tips but can definitely help. Also eating at the same time every day and going to sleep/waking up at the same time can help you regulate hormones better and fire up your metabolism.

9. "Any tips for targeting belly fat?"

Focusing on total body fitness is key—there's no magic exercise for belly fat. But reducing stress and getting enough sleep can specifically help with abdominal fat. It's about the big picture, not just crunches.

10. "What if I'm not seeing results fast enough?"

Think of it as a long race, not a quick one. Be happy about the wins that don't involve the scale, like feeling more powerful, sleeping more soundly, or noticing your clothes fit differently. Sometimes things don't go as planned, but being resilient means getting back up and trying again. Make sure you have cheerleaders, whether they're friends or family members.

CONCLUSION

Starting a health and fitness adventure is all about you, your body, what you want, and your life. If you have an endomorph body type, which means you might find it a bit harder to lose weight but super rewarding when you do, this journey is especially for you.

First off, we learned all about what being an endomorph means, like what makes you awesome and what challenges you might face. Setting goals that make sense for you is super important to keep your adventure on track. This book will dive into the best food and workout plans that help endomorphs like you stay healthy and fit in a way that works.

For eating, it's all about picking meals that keep you happy and full, and that help your body use energy better. Hope the 28-day plan helped you!

Exercise-wise, mixing things like lifting weights, doing cardio, and stretching is the secret sauce for building muscle, losing fat, and feeling more energetic. I am sure you loved the 12-week plan

Plus, we can't forget about taking breaks, chilling out, and making sure your brain is as healthy as your body.

In the end, this isn't just about beating the challenges of being an endomorph. It's about knowing what you've got and getting better every day without comparing yourself to others. Endomorphs can totally transform their health with the right info, attitude, and hard work. If you're ready to lead your own health adventure, this book is a beacon of hope and a practical companion.

So, let's not call this the end. It's just the start of a lifelong promise to stay healthy and fit. This is your chance to show what being healthy and fit really means, leading the charge for others walking the same path.

Printed in France by Amazon
Brétigny-sur-Orge, FR